Goddess Magic

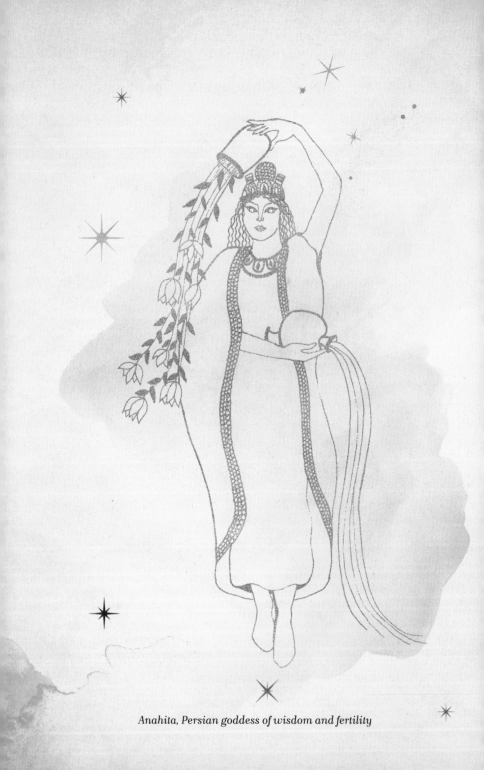

Anahita, Persian goddess of wisdom and fertility

Goddess Magic

A HANDBOOK OF SPELLS, CHARMS, AND RITUALS DIVINE IN ORIGIN

AURORA KANE

WELLFLEET PRESS

For my mother—an original Mother Goddess—and
to all my goddess friends and the goddess in us all

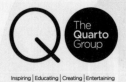

Brimming with creative inspiration, how-to projects, and useful information to enrich your everyday life, quarto.com is a favorite destination for those pursuing their interests and passions.

Inspiring | Educating | Creating | Entertaining

First published in 2022 by Wellfleet Press, an imprint of The Quarto Group,
142 West 36th Street, 4th Floor, New York, NY 10018, USA
T (212) 779-4972 F (212) 779-6058 www.Quarto.com

Wellfleet titles are also available at discount for retail, wholesale, promotional, and bulk purchase. For details, contact the Special Sales Manager by email at specialsales@quarto.com or by mail at The Quarto Group, Attn: Special Sales Manager, 100 Cummings Center Suite 265D, Beverly, MA 01915 USA.

10 9 8 7 6 5 4 3

ISBN: 978-1-57715-237-8

Library of Congress Control Number: 2021944788

Illustrations by Sosha Davis: page 2, 8, 22, 30, 34, 54, 58, 72, 76, 92, 95, 102, 105, 114, 117, 128, 146, 151, 153, 161, 208

Publisher: Rage Kindelsperger
Managing Editor: Cara Donaldson
Creative Director: Laura Drew
Editors: Leeann Moreau and Elizabeth You
Cover Illustration: Sosha Davis
Interior Design: Laura Klynstra

Printed in China

Contents

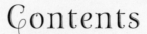

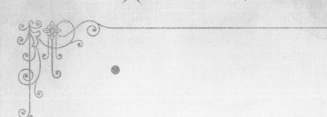

Step proudly into this sacred space we call the Goddess Realm,
To claim your place among the storied women who do roam
Among us here on Earth as well above, and so below,
To teach us, guide us, stand beside us, give us room to grow.

Their powers rule the realms of life we honor and hold dear,
Their wisdom whispers in our ear the words that calm our fears.
Their charms are offered freely—their beauty draws you near,
For once your magic binds with theirs, you'll join your goddess peers.

Discover what the goddesses have known for years on end—
That magic lies within your heart—its fire yours to tend.

Join hand in hand to form a circle with these goddess friends
To honor all who came before and those whom life portends.
For power shared does multiply and magic it does grow
When all are honored for their truth, their blazing flame does glow.

Introduction

Welcome to a celebration of feminine energy. Goddess magic is just that—as well as a chance to connect and learn from our ancestors and other powerful female figures who came before. Goddess magic allows us to get to know ourselves better along the way and tap into our divine goddess powers for doing good in the world and living our true, authentic lives.

The origins of the goddesses' importance in society, whether for worship or tales told to explain the everyday unexplainable occurrences, date back tens of thousands of years. She was at once mother, healer, animal, warrior, midwife, spring rain, autumn harvest, rainbow, and beautiful temptress—to cite but a few of her impressive accomplishments.

As you explore these 61 goddesses of many cultures and realms of influence presented here, you'll find those that can help with all matters of life, such as motherhood, love, success, strength, devotion, beauty, creativity, and healing. We'll seek each goddess's wisdom and guidance and learn her specific powers and favored offerings. With 45 spells and rituals to get you started, we'll honor these goddesses and heighten the energies we connect with to manifest intentions and live a meaningful and abundant life.

Along the way, you'll sharpen your intuition and feel more confident in your influence in the world than ever before. You'll feel magic everywhere and know how to fearlessly harness the energy for your needs and desires. You'll learn to tap into your inner goddess and release your magic into the world to make it a better place for all.

Instant goddess status is yours. No special magical experience or tools are required to enter this sacred realm. All that you need is within you, for that is where magic begins.

As with all things magic, though, the base is a connection to Nature and living in harmony with her natural rhythms. Do no harm, ever, and claim responsibility for your actions. Get ready to experience the divine magic working within your life.

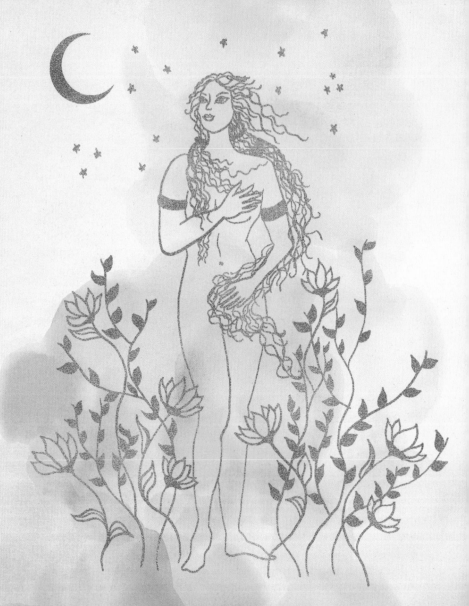

Venus, Roman goddess of love

Goddess Magic

The goddess as mother figure, the one who gave birth to all, speaks to the beginnings of reverence for the goddess—and all goddesses are an echo of her. She represents the cycles of life—birth and death, waxing and waning—and thus her close association, too, with the Moon.

As a spiritual figure of worship, the goddess grew in importance as societies became more agricultural. The ability of the land to bear crops and the fertility of Earth, as Great Mother, were paramount. Seeking her favor and celebrating her abundance had real meaning in people's lives as food needs were met—or not—seemingly on a whim.

But this life-giving figure is not just about childbirth or the harvest; she also gave life to the arts, crafts, healing, Nature, law and order, and more. And, in addition to being mother, she also became wife, seer, queen, judge, lover, homemaker, warrior, healer, and more. She rules the Sun and Moon, Earth and Sky. She is power in all its feminine forms and beauty.

There is much to learn from these wise women, and their magical energies come in all manner of influence. Key to these magical connections is belief—in the Universe, in the unseen, and in yourself.

Selecting a goddess, or two or three, to work with is the first step. Learning how to establish a relationship with her and align with her energies to release your intentions follows. Read on to discover more about goddess energy and how best to receive and use it.

GODDESS ENERGY

There is a vibrational energy innate in all things physical (trees, crystals, colors, people, etc.) and nonphysical (emotions, thoughts, music, sound, etc.). The law of the Universe tells us that with intentional direction and use of these energies, we can effect the change that we desire.

Drawing goddess energy into your magical practice serves to enhance your connection to the Universe. With magical energies deriving from all matter in Nature, goddesses add an ethereal, spiritual essence that speaks directly to the soul. They are the representation of the energy we seek to enhance our magic work. Channeling goddess energy gives us confidence to stand in our own place, speak our own words, and believe we can manifest what's in our heart. Our energies combined with goddess energies equal a powerful force for those who believe. But, as with all things magic, the intent must be true, and our hearts must be patient.

Although it's common for those practicing Wicca, also referred to as the goddess movement, to work with and alongside a number of goddesses to draw from their energy and wisdom, no specific belief system is required to benefit from goddess magic—it is open to all who believe.

DRAWING ON GODDESS ENERGY

Goddess energy is all around us—and within us as part of our own inner goddess. Drawing on this energy to weave it into ritual and spellwork starts with slowing down so we can recognize it. In the fast-paced, uncertain, out-of-control circumstances that we face today, it's as important as ever to practice self-care so we can thrive and grow. Connecting to our inner goddess and drawing on goddess magic can be part of that practice. In all, goddess energy feeds, reflects, and reinforces our divine feminine power. While this energy is sometimes sidelined, but never absent, we can boost it and connect with the Goddess Realm.

BEFRIENDING THE GODDESSES

To identify which goddess(es) can be most helpful to you and which might resonate with you most strongly, it's helpful to be open-minded and curious. Here are some ways to discover your new goddess besties.

- Research and learn all you can about the specific goddesses that call to you. This is the best way to know whether you've chosen the right goddess aligned with your energy and purpose. Or a goddess may choose you—research her, too, to understand why. You might also have an intuition of which goddess or goddesses may suit you. That's fine. Establish a relationship. Get to know her as you would any new friend.

- Set up an altar (see page 12), or multiple altars. An altar can be all-purpose, the artifacts and decorations changing with the seasons or your intentions; it can also be goddess specific, or intention specific.

- Meditate with your favorites, or invite some unfamiliar goddesses to sit with you in meditation, especially on specific issues where they can help.

- Journal with the goddesses for creativity, insight, problem solving, or any reason you desire.

- Make goddess offerings to seek favor, or sacrifices to create space for goddess magic to happen. They can be goddess specific or intention specific, as your circumstances require.

- Pray to your goddess for divine wisdom and guidance and be open to what you receive.

- Take a walk and connect with Nature.

- Show gratitude for blessings bestowed.

- Stay true to yourself and your dreams.

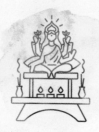

Creating Your Goddess Altar

Creating goddess magic does not require any special tools. In fact, the only necessary tool is *you* and the magical belief you have in connecting with Universal energies to influence outcomes. That said, some tools can be fun to create and use in your magical practice, such as an altar, to inspire your work and manifest the vibrational energy you'll use to release intentions into the Universe.

An altar defines your sacred space and provides a visual reminder and a physical presence—inside or outside, when working in groups or alone—to focus your energy, meditate, or try a goddess spell or two.

Your altar does not have to be fancy and can be as simple as a windowsill—or even a cardboard box, for an altar to go! It can be a shelf, bookshelf, or tabletop, too, where you display your goddess statues and candles, crystals, or other reminders of your intentions to keep you aware every day of the work you're doing and your priorities.

You may even decide to have more than one altar—each honoring a different goddess, or changing with the seasons as your life's intentions grow and evolve. You can also create altars reflecting specific intentions: Set up an altar in your bedroom that is devoted to attracting love; one in the kitchen to boost energies for raising a healthy family; one in a quiet corner for cultivating gratitude or gathering strength, for example. Maybe you'll create one dedicated to a sacred Moon goddess or your ancestors. Set up an altar outside to celebrate Nature and her goddesses, along with the charms and abundance she lends to your world. Be as fancy, creative, or minimalist as you like.

Physically cleaning the space where your altar resides removes negative energy and makes room for good vibes to flourish. Wipe it clean with rosemary water or rose water. Sweep it clean with a bundle of lavender blooms. Ceremonially cleaning your space can be an alternative; consider a besom broom or common sage cleansing spray to help whisk away any energy that does not serve.

Your altar represents you—your heart, hopes, dreams, intentions, and life. If you stay true to your heart, your altar will be ready to help you work your magic when called upon.

What to Place on Your Altar

Your altar will evolve along with your magical practice. Decorating your altar is a personal choice. Cover it with a cloth if you wish—maybe in a color that represents your intentions or the goddess you're evoking. As much as possible, keep the elements that make up your altar natural, for their innate, individual energies. On your altar, you may wish to include any or all of the following, but always do what feels right to you and is true to your heart:

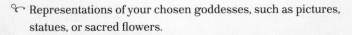

- ⌁ Representations of your chosen goddesses, such as pictures, statues, or sacred flowers.

- ⌁ Water—whether charged by the Full Moon's light or sourced from a river, stream, or ocean—for cleansing and blessing your altar.

- A bowl of clean soil, Himalayan salt, crystals, or seeds to represent the element of Earth and all you admire and worship there.

- Candles in colors that support your intentions (see page 15), or use colored crystal candleholders with white candles in their place.

- Crystals whose vibrational energies connect with your goals and resonate with you.

- Essential oils to incorporate into spellwork or rituals, or for use in meditation.

- Pictures of loved ones, or other reminders of those important to you.

- Goddess or tarot cards, rune tiles, a small cauldron, a scrying bowl, or other tools to assist in daily meditation, intention setting, or spellwork.

- Dried herbs, fresh flowers, or other plants to reflect your intentions and add an element of natural beauty to celebrate and magnify the energies your soul seeks.

- Books that have special meaning, including a journal.

- Bells, chimes, or a singing bowl.

CALLING ON THE GODDESSES

When calling on the goddesses, and to define your purpose for consulting with them, working in a sacred space, such as on an altar, can be helpful. This is a time of quiet, calm, and inner focus. Visualize the goddess as she appears to you. Visualize your intentions and the outcome desired. Ask her to join you and ask for her help. Provide an offering of goodwill or thanks and close your ceremony with an expression of gratitude.

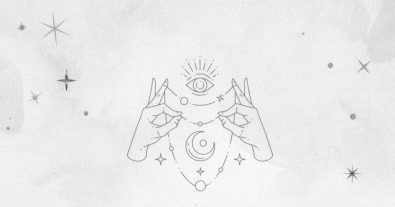

WORKING WITH GODDESS ENERGY

Goddess energy surrounds you and is available to you at any time.
Working with goddess energy is as simple as asking or waiting for a
goddess to choose you—and the time that she'll make herself known.
When you're ready, send your request to the Universe and be ready to
receive her response.

Once you've found your perfect goddess, work with her—through
intention setting, meditating, journaling, or acts of kindness in her
honor—and her energy to manifest intentions and bring goddess
magic into your life. In addition to these tools, use others that resonate
with you and bring meaning to your life, such as poetry, music, dance,
crystal work, and more.

INTENTION SETTING

All action springs from intention—and intentions, like all things, are
made of energy, which connects us universally. This energy is the
reason we can unite so powerfully with goddess energy to multiply our
magic and influence what we manifest. Setting clear intentions is one of
the first steps in goddess magic.

To define your intentions, consider: What do you seek? What do
you need? What do you wish? What needs attention in your life? Reach
deep into your soul to acknowledge, without fear or judgment, what is
important to you and what will make you truly happy. Call upon an
allied goddess to absorb her energy and lessons to bring clarity to
your thoughts.

Setting specific intentions based on these self-defined priorities creates goals aligned with your values and dreams. Defining intentions keeps us focused and living in the present, and can help improve our overall well-being. Important, too, is living mindfully without judgment, learning to accept what is, and working to change circumstances, as we desire.

Remember that intentions change as we change. Don't be afraid to adjust, replace, or refine them as your needs and priorities evolve. Stay true to yourself and your goddess power in seeking your dreams and desires.

Is Anyone Listening?

When you release your intentions into the Universe, the vibrational energy ripples cause chain reactions that can take time to reveal themselves. Results may be delayed—or not what you expected—but likely are there if you look and listen carefully.

If, however, you really feel your intentions, along with your inner goddess, are being sidelined:

- Be clear. Are your energy signals confusing? Do you know what's in your heart? Be honest, nonjudgmental, accepting, and realistic in your assessment. You cannot raise your vibrational energy if your actions are in misalignment with your heart.

- Be consistent. Focus on what's important.

- Be attuned. Review your timing and assess your energy levels.

- Be patient and believe. Magic won't be hurried.

- Be present. Acknowledge what's around you and cultivate a grateful heart as you work toward your desired goals.

- Be kind to the goddesses. Perhaps a goddess offering is in order?

- Be kind to yourself—engage in mindful meditation (see page 17) or other self-care rituals that make you feel like the goddess you are. Forgive yourself and others.

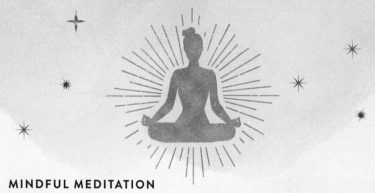

MINDFUL MEDITATION

Another useful tool in harnessing goddess energy is mindful meditation. This type of meditation offers the chance to slow down and reflect, to invite the goddess to be with you and to be able to tap into her wisdom while exploring your inner thoughts and feelings, which can then become intentions set to achieve your goals.

To meditate, in general, is to engage in contemplation or reflection, or to engage in a mental exercise (as in concentrating on your breathing or repeating a mantra) in order to reach a heightened level of spiritual awareness. Buddhists, who have been practicing meditation for millennia, believe it develops concentration, clarity, emotional positivity, and a calmness that is needed to see the truth. When you focus your thoughts, you eliminate the endless lists running through your brain that may be causing you stress or worry, or that are making it hard to focus and make decisions.

Mindful meditation is the practice of being present, where you strive for an increased awareness of being in the moment, without preconceived notions or judgment, and paying attention to yourself—your breathing, emotions, sensations, and thoughts. Meditation is not about tuning out everything in our lives but, rather, tuning in to the present and being with ourselves.

For those today who practice meditation, it is commonly a way to relieve stress and reduce anxiety. If you've been meditating for a while, you have already experienced the positive things it can bring to your life. If not, you have nothing to lose; there is no right or wrong, and it doesn't have to take lots of time.

Regular meditation can bring about a transforming sense of relaxation and ease. Learning to focus your thoughts helps clear the clutter that can accumulate in our brains. It helps us to see what matters most and, more importantly, just to be for a while. Meditation has been said to contribute to overall improved physical and mental well-being, including helping develop a new perspective on stressful situations, reducing negative emotions and reactions, boosting creativity, fostering acceptance, decreasing pain, and increasing happiness. Meditation can also help develop your intuitive senses, which are helpful for all your magical work.

You don't need a lot of, or really any, fancy equipment or gear to meditate—only a quiet space (outdoors surrounded by Nature is a great option), a comfortable position, and an open mind—and maybe a gentle alarm if you prefer to time your sessions. Make this as fancy as you like, with essential oils, crystals, candles, other rituals, etc., or as simple as just breathing.

Mindful meditation takes practice and consistency—even 10 minutes a day can help—but once you begin to feel the benefits in your life, you will crave the quiet peace that meditation affords. Whatever you choose to make it, make it regular and stress-free.

Goddess Meditation Basics

~ Find a quiet, comfortable place where you won't be disturbed. Relax. Set a gentle alarm if you wish to time your session.

~ Close your eyes, if you are comfortable doing so, to limit visual distractions.

~ Ask. Invite a specific goddess to join you, or let one select you. Visualize her entering your space, sitting with you, walking with you, comforting you. What is she telling you? How do you feel?

~ Breathe. Bring your attention to your breathing. Breathe in and out through your nose, naturally yet fully. Focus your attention on each in-breath and out-breath; feel your body grow on the in-breath and feel it collapse on the out-breath. Feel your breath calming and centering the energy within you—let yourself relax.

~ Imagine each inhale fills you with goddess wisdom and love— from top to bottom—cleansing and clearing any negativity, hurt, or fear.

- ∿ Visualize your exhale taking with it anything causing you pain, as you replace it on the inhale with soothing kindness and infinite power.

- ∿ Focus. As you concentrate on your breath, your mind may wander. Gently acknowledge it and return your focus to your breath. Listen to the goddess within. Alternatively, as you continue your breathing you may scan your body, focusing your attention solely on one part before moving on to the next—starting at your toes and moving upward to your scalp. If a particular body part feels tense or painful, focus your mind and breathing on that part until it is relaxed, then move on to the next. Again, if your attention wanders, gently refocus and continue the process.

- ∿ Be grateful. When your timer sounds, or you are ready, return your focus to your surroundings. Open your eyes. Wiggle your toes. Take a moment to give thanks to the goddess for the quiet time and be grateful for the space that welcomes you before returning to your normal activities—charged with goddess energy that both soothes and inspires.

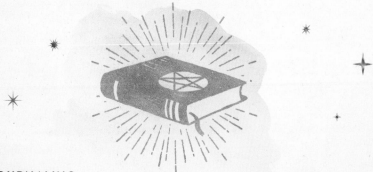

JOURNALING

Another way to tap into goddess wisdom is with journaling. Whatever you desire to manifest, putting your intentions into writing—whether in a diary, journal, calendar, or other volume—creates a record to serve as a reminder as well as one you can reflect on and check in on for progress along the way. Putting things in writing, in general, moves us from the "thought" stage to the "action" stage. It keeps you committed, motivated, focused, reminded. It frees up space in your brain for other things. It keeps you grateful and honest. It can reduce stress. Writing about your dreams and intentions creates another form of energy to release your thoughts into the Universe.

When journaling with the goddesses, you may want to journal about issues and intentions specific to a goddess you're working with, or journal about everyday issues and intentions and let the goddess energy work through you in the way that feels most natural.

- Journal after meditating, especially if with a goddess. What did you learn? What do you still need to know? What surprised you?

- Write about your inner goddess needs and desires.

- Decorate your journal with drawings or images, poetry or spells that evoke your goddess.

- Write down questions you wish to explore with your goddess or record times you felt her presence, including where you were and what you were doing. How did you know she was with you? Let your writing channel her message.

- Imagine yourself as the goddess and write about your special powers. Write freely and honestly—without judgment.

- Create affirmations that channel goddess energy.

- Journal about spells and rituals you've tried and created, and record their results.

- Journal daily or only as needed, but make space in your life to let the magic in.

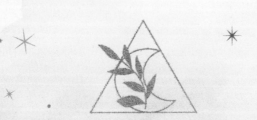

TO INVOKE OR EVOKE THE GODDESS

When discussing communication with the goddesses, "invocation" and "evocation" are similar terms but deliver different results in the magical world. For those with much experience in their magical practice, there is a difference and that can include how one prepares to invite the spirit goddess in and for what purpose.

To "invoke" a goddess is to call her forth, to call upon her, often with an incantation, to communicate and establish a relationship. Invocation may involve a ritual or offering. In essence, you invite the goddess into your home and life—almost as if she's stepping into your shoes. Drawing down the Moon is a classic example.

To "evoke" a goddess is to conjure her spirit, to bring to your mind, to ask her to work beside and with you for a specific purpose and outcome. Think of it as more task oriented, where she may then be thanked and released from duty when the job is done.

Depending on circumstances and intentions, you may do either. However, be advised it is best to invoke or evoke only one goddess at a time, so choose wisely based on your needs, intentions, and feelings about the goddess.

Let's explore the Goddess Realm. As we start our journey, remember:

- ᕗ *Honor your goddess within—and the goddess within each other.*
- ᕗ *Honor the goddess you choose, or the one who chooses you, with offerings and gratitude.*
- ᕗ *Honor the Earth as Nature goddess. Honor the Moon as Mother goddess.*
- ᕗ *Believe in your goddess power.*

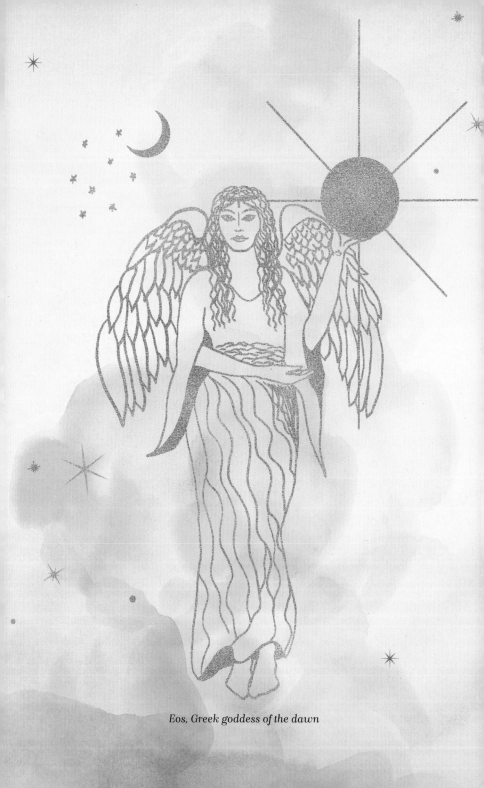

Eos, Greek goddess of the dawn

Goddesses of
Love and Beauty

The goddesses who were worshipped for love and their beauty were extraordinary creatures who possessed self-confidence, independence, and awareness of their sexuality and sensuality, as well as great passion and pride. Their beauty, in a sense, radiates from their core and is a reflection of all around them. They can teach us about many things—not just physical beauty, for as they say, that is in the eye of the beholder. These ladies were also fierce protectors, trusted confidantes, and worthy partners and possessed strong personalities.

Able to light our lives with their mere presence, they can help us feel youthful in body, mind, and spirit; beautiful; and hopeful—with the ease and confidence that come with those traits. They promise the unending joy of romance and love and offer the strength to withstand its failings. They can help us refine our independent spirits and honor our intentions. Pamper your inner goddess as much as you need to feel adored. While decidedly feminine, their spirits are fierce and courageous.

They are sure of their place in the world and their influence on it, so don't be shy about seeking their help and guidance.

CELEBRATE THE GODDESS

Rejoice in your newfound friendships and celebrate the goddess. Honor her special days, work with her symbols, or just better appreciate her point of view with these tips and facts.

Eos (Greek) / Aurora (Roman) / Tesana (Etruscan), page 25

This Greek goddess appears in literature more than any other. Read stories about her! Get up early and appreciate the beauty of the dawn.

Freya (Norse), page 26

Freya loved jewelry, with her most cherished piece being the Brisingamen necklace, made by and earned from the dwarfs. Wear your best jewelry when working with Freya.

Hebe (Greek) / Juventas (Roman), page 27

Hebe's chalice with which she served nectar to the gods was exquisitely decorated. Dust off your most cherished china cup or other decorative vessel for your next toast to Hebe.

Inanna (Sumerian/Mesopotamian), page 28

Closely associated with the morning and evening star: revel in their beauty when seeking Inanna's company.

Venus (Roman) / Aphrodite (Greek), page 29

August 12 is the day to honor Venus; the fourth day of each month is sacred to Aphrodite: make your offerings appropriately.

When beauty floats upon the air, we recognize its scent...

for love ensues, each breath we take, a gift that's goddess-sent.

Unable to resist your face, my goddess of delight, you sing of beauty all around—reflecting hope and light.

When passions stir and romance blooms, don't hesitate to fall straight in the arms of goddess love—her beauty beckons all.

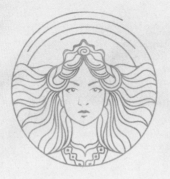

EOS (GREEK) / AURORA (ROMAN) /
TESANA (ETRUSCAN)

Sister of Helios, the Sun god, and Selene, the Moon goddess, Eos—Titan goddess of the dawn —makes her presence felt each day. She radiates intense beauty, which shines bright with possibilities. Mother of the winds and the Evening Star, Eos represents sexuality, fertility, youth, beauty, hope, and passion. She is a natural leader, as she ushers the Sun from night to day, sweeping across the sky in her golden chariot powered by winged horses. Beware her persistent desire and pursuit of new relationships, indicating dissatisfaction and an unawareness of self in what makes her happy.

Call on Eos for guidance in matters of romance and fertility. Seek her company when hope fades and darkness begins to overtake your spirit.

POWERS

Eos brings us light each day—announcing the arrival of fertile new opportunities. She holds great wisdom and an ability to banish evil spirits. When working with this goddess, pursue honesty in relationships as well as with yourself.

OFFERINGS

Saffron is sacred to her and her glorious robes were dyed with the spice; described as the rosy fingers of dawn; crystals or candles in any dawn-related colors—pink/rose, orange/peach, blue/lavender, yellow/gold—are adored.

FREYA (NORSE)

No ordinary goddess, Freya, whose name means "lady," held a significant and powerful position in the Goddess Realm. She was revered for her beauty and is goddess of love, wealth, fertility, and war, among other things, and teacher of magic, including the valuable knowledge of the runes. Here, we focus on her as goddess of love. Though she is married to Odr, he is frequently away in battle or on other kingdom business, leaving Freya to fend for herself. Her stunning beauty makes her the object of much attention and fidelity is not her strong suit. As Freya is the goddess of love, she embraces a sexual love, and she shares it willingly—even trading sex with four dwarfs for her most favored piece of jewelry, a beautiful amber necklace. Freya also loves to travel and is well equipped to do so: choosing from a cat-pulled chariot, a magical cloak of feathers with which she can fly undetected through the skies, or a wild boar as a mount.

Seek Freya's inspiration when charting your course and stand tall in honor of who you are. Invoke Freya in all your spellwork, as she is an eager teacher and will guide your ways.

POWERS

Freya's sexual favors gave her bargaining power—and she was a woman who knew what she wanted and was not afraid to go after it. Her mastery of magic, which she taught freely, included the ability to influence the fate and fortunes of others, for which she was enormously respected. Her independent spirit helped her carve her own path.

OFFERINGS

Jewelry, especially amber, is a welcome gift to Freya, as are honey, flowers—especially roses—strawberries, and all things cat related. Travel-related items, such as maps, and feathers to adorn her altar, are favored as well. Runes tiles, with which to engage Freya, are also a fun idea.

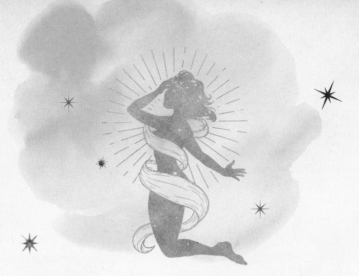

HEBE (GREEK) / JUVENTAS (ROMAN)

Hebe, goddess of youth, was among the most beautiful of the goddesses. Although it is easy to see how anyone could fall in love with her, it was her famed ability to restore youth—and, thus it was thought, to dispel all one's troubles—that caused others to search her out for her great gift. She also tended the Olympian gods as cupbearer, serving nectar and ambrosia as they pleased.

Call on Hebe when a youthful outlook might give you some new perspective. Youth is a state of mind to be embraced with the wisdom that comes with age.

POWERS

Hebe's greatest power was restoring eternal youth and beauty to those who had aged. She sometimes required convincing that the request was worthy of granting, which tells us she may have been wise beyond her years.

OFFERINGS

Place your gifts to Hebe in a cup, a most appropriate vessel for her to receive them. Wine (nectar) and sweets (ambrosia) will bring her favor. Fresh flowers placed on your altar are also a lovely way to honor her youth and beauty, as are perfumes.

INANNA (SUMERIAN/MESOPOTAMIAN)

One of the oldest goddesses on record, the powerful Inanna, who worked her way up from simple goddess of vegetation to goddess of heaven, ruled over beauty, love, fertility, and war. She later became known as Ishtar and was also identified with Diana/Artemis and Aphrodite, among other goddesses. Her provocative nature leaves us multiple tales of her sexual abilities, and she was as fierce about love as about war—another of her supreme realms.

In her quest for more power, Inanna used her feminine wiles fully to steal the gifts of the arts, music, and wisdom from the god Enki, which she used to educate and cultivate her patron city of Uruk. A lion is frequently by her side, suggesting a courageous spirit who inspired fierce loyalty.

With her ability to handle well the typically feminine aspects of love as well as the masculine territory of war, she was a complex being and very much a reflection of today's independent women.

Call on Inanna for any aspect of love and family where a combination of heart and reason will serve you well.

POWERS

Inanna's powers are vast and potent. Inanna's beauty and charm make her easy to get to know and her powers of war and wisdom make her hard to forget. Her courage can be an inspiration and her independence sparks action. She can awaken the desire within that is needed for issues of fertility in all areas, bringing seeds from germination to fruition.

OFFERINGS

Offer Inanna a beautifully decorated altar upon which you can place figs and apples, wine, lapis lazuli, and sweet baked goods. Add music to honor her gift. Place seeds in a dish on your altar to represent fertility and germination, whether into children, plants, ideas, or other things needed to be brought to fruition. Plant a vegetable garden in her honor, or a simple potted herb to tend—parsley for fertility, or perhaps thyme for courage. The Empress tarot card is especially attuned to working with this goddess.

VENUS (ROMAN) / APHRODITE (GREEK)

Venus, Aphrodite to the Greeks, was the Roman goddess of passionate love, sexuality, beauty, abundance, fertility—and seduction. She is said to be born of the sea, so water is a powerful element and symbol of Venus and our feminine side, which we all have. Water is life-giving and nurturing, offering emotion and fluidity, calming intuition. Married to Vulcan, she bore him no children, but her fertility was borne out by numerous children from multiple lovers—both gods and mortals—who could not resist her tantalizing energies. So beautiful, in fact, was she that virtually all were said to be unable to resist her. A face like an angel hid the passions of her soul. She embraces pleasure in all its forms and is eager to help us experience all life has to offer. Venus is honored in April as the fertile Earth awakens and blooms.

Call upon Venus when your desire is to ignite or rekindle passionate love in your relationship, or to nurture your burning inner passion. Emulate her sensuality and charm. Seek her guidance on looking your best and her confidence to reveal your enchanting beauty to the world to attract what you desire.

POWERS

Venus, through time, has been goddess of many things, but passion—for love and the ability to attract lovers, and for life—is her most famously celebrated one. And, perhaps as an allied power, Venus could tame the wildest of animals. She had power over Nature and shines as the brightest star in the sky. Born from the sea, she is also a revered protector of sailors. Her powers of charm and seduction are the stuff of legend.

OFFERINGS

As a goddess of great beauty, Venus will be pleased with gorgeous fresh flowers, especially roses. Other meaningful offerings are seashells, seasonal fruits, honey, and anything red—the color of passionate love—such as red candles or garnets. Keeping her altar tended will keep Venus's fire alive in your soul.

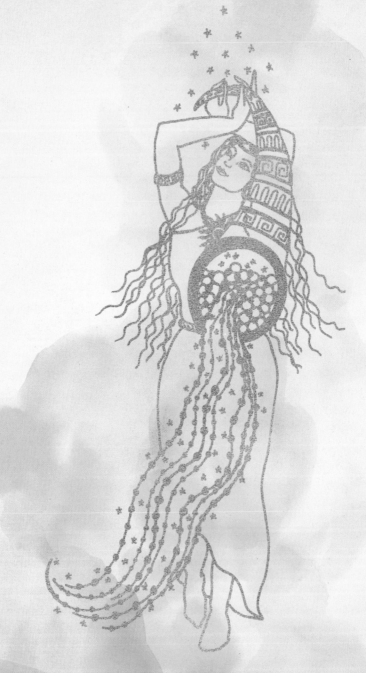

Fortuna, Roman goddess of luck and prosperity

Goddesses of Marriage, Fertility, and Motherhood

The Mother Goddess is a figure known and revered by numerous cultures and belief systems, and in pagan and Wiccan traditions is an aspect of the Triple Goddess.

Like most mothers, she is a complex figure—at once loving, nurturing, wise, fearsome, independent, feisty, and, sometimes, unpredictable. She also shares characteristics and responsibilities with goddesses of Earth in matters of fertility, creation, growth, and abundance and goddesses of hearth and home in all matters domestic; she is typically the personification of Nature itself. And, like all mothers everywhere, her job is multifaceted and never-ending, so you may connect with other goddesses whose powers are allied.

These adored goddesses offer help with fertility, with an ease that can germinate in all areas of your life, and childbirth wishes. They serve as role models of wife and mother, who can be called on for a variety of family needs and circumstances. Remember, mothers are wise beyond their years as they trust their intuition implicitly.

When seeking the company of these goddesses, work their influence into your journaling, ritual work, or spellwork, or just call on them in the moment to keep you grounded. Offerings are encouraged, but mothers love thanks and gratitude above all.

CELEBRATE THE GODDESS

Rejoice in your newfound friendships and celebrate the goddess. Honor her special days, work with her symbols, or just appreciate her point of view more with these tips and facts.

Corn Mother (Native American), page 35

The Sabbat festival Lammas on August 1, the first of three harvest Sabbats, celebrates the early harvest and Corn Mother, as well as Ceres (see below). Bake bread and share with friends.

Cybele (Phrygian), page 36

March 25 is a day designated to honor Cybele. As the pine tree is sacred to her, gather pine cones and make a wreath for your altar. Sprinkle pine nuts on a salad and give thanks for Cybele's bounty.

Danu (Celtic), page 38

The Sabbat festival of Beltane on May 1, or May Day, celebrates Danu. Spring's peak is about to burst into summer's abundance. Plant a garden in honor of Danu or tend to the seeds of new intentions.

Demeter (Greek) / Ceres (Roman), page 39

As with Corn Mother, Lammas marks the celebration of Demeter; April 12–19 sees the festival Cerealia, in honor of Ceres. Make a cake to mark the occasion.

Hera (Greek) / Juno (Roman), page 41

Hera is frequently pictured holding a pomegranate. Sprinkle its seeds on a salad, enjoy the juice in a cocktail, or fill a bowl with their beauty to adorn your kitchen table.

Isis (Egyptian), page 43

Frequently depicted wearing the horns of a cow, Isis is celebrated at the vernal equinox, about March 20, as life returns to Earth. Add a splash of milk to your coffee or tea and thank Isis for her wisdom and powerful magic.

Mawu (West African), page 45

Mawu soothes the African continent by bringing cooler weather. She is celebrated during winter solstice (Yule), generally December 21, a time of celebration and offerings—make yours under the Full Moon in her honor.

Ninhursag (Sumerian, Mesopotamian), page 46

As Ninhursag is goddess of stones and rocky ground, a reading of the story "Stone Soup" is in order, or make a pot of soup as an offering—you may want to serve the stones on the side!

Oshun (African), page 47

The number five is sacred to Oshun. Using it and some other simple offerings, begin your day aligned with her spirit and carry her energies as you work to manifest dreams: Cut an orange into five pieces, dust your toast with cinnamon, and drizzle a bit of honey into your tea. Offer a quiet thanks for her gentle guidance and enjoy a breakfast made for a goddess.

Selene (Greek) / Luna (Roma), page 48

Selene is honored at the Full Moon. Her color is white, and Monday (Moon-day) is in her honor. Place a vase of fresh white flowers in your home each Monday if Selene's company is sought.

Triple Goddess, page 50

Reflect on the message of the Three of Cups tarot card to get closer to this complex goddess. Celebrate the generations in your family in honor of her three phases.

Yemaya (African), page 52

If you're a beach baby, you may feel a special connection to this water goddess as you swim within her embrace. Water signs Cancer, Scorpio, and Pisces are also attuned to her message. A fresh watermelon salad would be a lovely meal to celebrate her gifts and presence in your life.

O Mother Goddess who gives life,
in thankfulness I bow tonight.

With outstretched arms to honor you,
to sing the praise of all you do.

I ask your blessing of my life,
to love and marry—and breathe life

into the plans we've made today
to conquer fear and challenge strife.

To see the cycle start anew,
each precious gift is born of you.

The fruits of labor reaped this way engage
my soul and light the way.

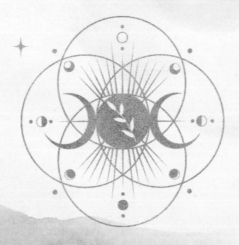

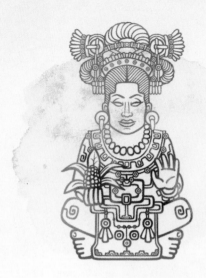

CORN MOTHER (NATIVE AMERICAN)

Like all goddesses, Corn Mother has influence over many areas: fertility, children, abundance, healing, fate, and more, and numerous stories of her abound. She is credited by Indigenous Native American agriculture tribes both as being the first woman and for giving birth to corn, with its life-sustaining nourishment and symbolism of sacred knowledge. Before Corn Mother died, she passed on the knowledge of planting and farming corn to her two sons—which included dragging her body through a field where corn sprung up in her path (a story for another time)—so that her legacy was reborn each year with the harvest. She is a mother symbol and goddess of fertility and abundance seen in many cultures and pantheons, and known, in concept, by many names, such as Demeter/Ceres, for example.

Call on Corn Mother to nourish you in any way that sustains.

POWERS

Corn Mother's selfless love is one of nourishment and acceptance. She is the mother we all know who feeds us constantly as a sign of her care and adoration. She readily shares all she has, including her wisdom, that we may lead productive lives.

OFFERINGS

Corn—in all its forms. Keep a dried ear of corn on your altar to channel Corn Mother's protective energies. Cornstalk dolls are a favorite. Fill your cauldron with clean soil and sprinkle some seeds on top as a gift to Corn Mother. Clean water and sunlight are also welcome, as they nurture the corn toward full growth.

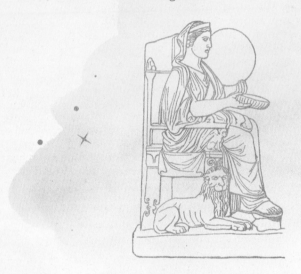

CYBELE (PHRYGIAN)

This ancient goddess, whose tale originated in ancient Phrygia, was called Magna Mater by the Romans, or Great Mother, and this universal mother figure is responsible for giving birth to all animals, Nature, and humanity. She is often pictured seated in a chariot pulled by two lions—a symbol of her powers of protection, or perhaps her fierce personality. Another legend tells of her origins as a forest witch, abandoned at birth and raised by the lions who found her. Unlike other goddesses of her time, she was protected by a group of priests, the Galli, comprising castrated eunuchs.

Legend says Cybele fell in love with Attis, a beautiful young shepherd boy, but Attis chose another for his wife. So enraged by jealousy was Cybele that she disrupted his wedding, driving Attis insane and into the woods, where he was found lying dead (self-castrated!) near a pine tree. Instantly remorseful, Cybele pleaded to Zeus, who decreed that Cybele could bring him back to life and declared the pine tree sacred.

Work with Cybele for all things divine, feminine, and anything associated with children, healing, and powers of a woman's intuition—but beware her jealous tendencies.

POWERS

Cybele's powers are those of the most complex mother you can imagine! She is associated with healing, protection, childbirth, and motherhood, and the cycle of life, death, and rebirth. Cybele's wisdom and compassion can be of great influence in times of joy and of sorrow. She is a patient teacher and fierce protector.

OFFERINGS

Music—especially of cymbals and drums—honey, fruit, roses, pine cones, pine essential oil, natural crystals or rocks, or other elements of Earth make meaningful offerings to Cybele.

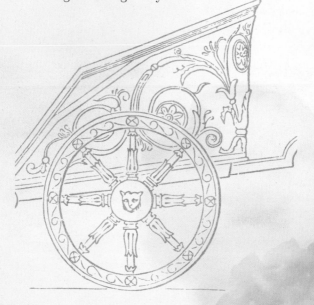

DANU (CELTIC)

Danu, which means "flowing," is the great Mother Goddess and a Triple Goddess. In ancient Irish tradition, she is the mother of all Irish gods, people, and the fairy people—descended from the Tuatha Dé Danann, the people of Danu—a disparate group of otherworldly magical folk she reunited and nurtured to great skill and strength. As earth goddess of land and water, Danu has influence over fertility, bounty, wisdom, wind, and rivers—and is credited with lending her name to the beautiful Danube River.

Call to Danu on the night of a Full Moon for her most powerful creative wisdom, or on the New Moon when new beginnings are desired.

POWERS

Danu brings us the comfort, love, and acceptance of a mother; the grounding of Earth; the wisdom of experience; the bounty of children and harvest; and the healing, soothing powers of water. Her powers of leadership and natural inclination toward teaching are key to the survival of the Tuatha Dé Danann. No matter the challenge, Danu does not back down or give up.

OFFERINGS

Stones, especially river stones, gifts of water, or anything blue—the color of water—flowers, apples, and any bounty of the Earth, really, will please Danu.

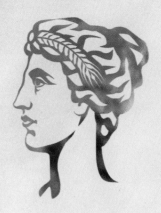

DEMETER (GREEK) / CERES (ROMAN)

Goddess of fertility in agriculture and the harvest, and law and order (arising from the transition to an agrarian society with defined living and planting areas), Demeter champions women, marriage, and health. She rules the seasons—from birth to death and rebirth. Ceres, appropriately, lends her name to cereal, from the grains of the harvest. Demeter is sometimes considered another expression of Corn Mother, as she is credited with teaching humans to tend the earth and grow and use corn crops.

Demeter's daughter, Persephone, was abducted by Hades and taken to his Underworld to be his wife. Her disappearance caused Demeter much suffering, which led her to abandon her goddess duties. The crops suffered, the people suffered, but Demeter remained in mourning. Hades, finally convinced by Zeus, agreed to release Persephone—but not without a compromise: She could return to Earth for part of the year (spring, summer, and autumn), spending the remaining time (winter) with Hades in the Underworld. Demeter is worshipped on Persephone's return in the spring and again on her departure in autumn.

Call on Demeter for her ability to relieve suffering, her wisdom in tending to the harvest, her undying mother's love, and when the transition of the seasons might bring on a change of mood that needs adjusting. She can also help restore a little law and order in your world, when things seem to be getting out of control, and assist in finding precious things that have been lost.

POWERS

Demeter's powers were in producing abundance, especially at the harvest, bestowing fertility that crops would grow and produce, and endurance. She ruled the seasons and weather. Demeter was also a shape-shifter, allowing her to blend in and fit into any situation to her advantage. And, as an Olympian, she had the ability to bless and curse at will, depending on how she felt about you at that moment!

OFFERINGS

Sacred plants to her were corn, wheat, and pumpkin. Bread is a simple offering. She is often pictured with a torch, lighting her search for Persephone, so candles in earth colors are meaningful to her. She will reject offerings of all flowers, as it was when her daughter was out picking them that she was abducted.

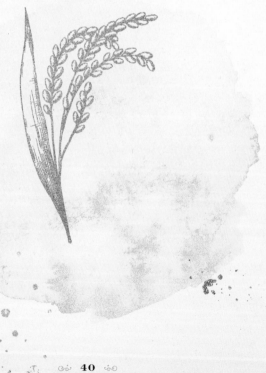

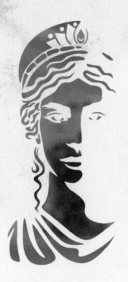

HERA (GREEK) / JUNO (ROMAN)

Wife of Zeus and queen of Olympus, the beautiful Hera represented the ideal female. She was goddess of marriage, birth, and family but possessed a mean, jealous streak. She also reigned over the skies and stars.

Though her husband strayed, Hera remained faithful to him and became the symbol of true fidelity (as well as a vengeful woman scorned). In a plot to kill Zeus, she stole his lightning bolt (!). The plot failed, so she turned her wrath on his lovers. Among Zeus's many lovers—and targets of Hera's jealousy—was the nymph Callisto (meaning "most beautiful"), who bore Zeus a son. Hera transformed Callisto into a bear that could be hunted by the goddess Artemis. Zeus, seeing what was developing, intervened and turned her into the constellation Ursa Major and placed his son in the sky as Ursa Minor.

Her Roman counterpart, Juno, was honored for her faithfulness in marriage and her nurturing care of her family. She did not possess the jealous qualities that Hera made famous. Juno lent her name to the month of June, a favorite time of year for weddings.

Call on Hera for all matters in the management of family issues, with fertility wishes, and to manifest wishes of marriage.

POWERS

As goddess of women and marriage, Hera has the power to bless or curse a union. As protector of women and children, Hera is often evoked to aid in childbirth, and her powers can also protect overall health. Her goddess power of eternal youth can be called upon when our own beauty feels lacking, and her aid will also restore self-esteem. She is strong under pressure and can bless you with blue skies as a reward and wisdom, when requested.

OFFERINGS

Appropriate offerings for Hera include the pomegranate, symbol of fertility, and pomegranate seeds; peacock feathers (imitation, of course!), as the peacock is sacred to her; the lily, a sacred flower; or any white flower. Burn a white candle in her honor.

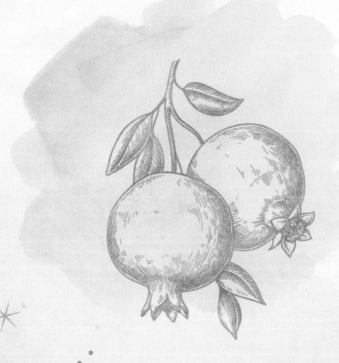

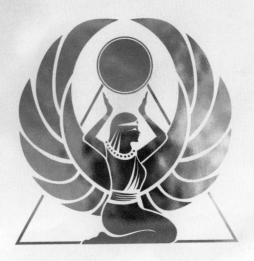

ISIS (EGYPTIAN)

Isis, whose name means "female of the throne," is also known as Lady of Ten Thousand Names, and she was a goddess extraordinaire. She was goddess of the Moon, marriage, mothers, fertility, and magic. She was also a healer and teacher and assumed the roles and responsibilities of other goddesses as her popularity and influence grew.

Isis rose to her supreme power by tricking Ra, god of the Sun, into revealing his secret password to unlock the power he held over life and death. She was sister-wife of Osiris and mother of Horus. Isis, with Osiris, ruled the gods until her jealous brother killed him. Unable to bear her loss, she used her magic gifts to bring Osiris back to life, and later to give him immortality. Isis is closely associated with the flooding of the Nile, caused by her unstoppable tears on the death of Osiris, and thus its fertility and ability to produce foods. She symbolized rebirth.

Call on Isis when her gifts of magic can help solve problems that seem insurmountable—especially to give yourself the upper hand. Invoke her to experience the joys of motherhood if fertility issues are of concern. Seek her counsel in child rearing and emulate her loyalty as a wife and mother.

POWERS

Isis was nothing if not ambitious and was honored as an excellent mother and loyal wife. She is not afraid to love bravely and feel deeply. Her generosity is legendary, as is her willingness to do what is needed to get what she wants. Her powers of persuasive speech earned her the sacred secrets to life and death.

OFFERINGS

Milk, honey, and flowers are traditional offerings to Isis. A spoken prayer of gratitude is a powerful gift as well.

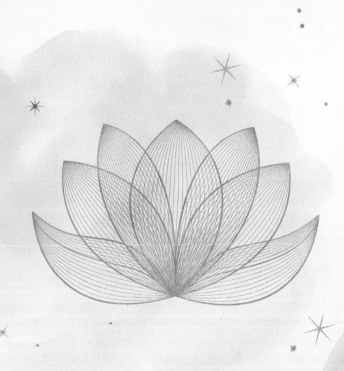

MAWU (WEST AFRICAN)

Mother Earth goddess Mawu is reflective of both the Sun and Moon. She is creator of all life, fashioning it from clay and water. She inspires passion, creative energy, birth, abundance, and the pregnant possibilities of hope.

Call on Mawu when you need help delivering new ideas into existence or when your burden feels too heavy to bear alone. When your feminine energies feel a bit sidelined, Mawu can get you back on track. Evoking Mawu when feeling centered and grounded will restore confidence in your convictions.

POWERS

Mawu offers the lessons of living in harmony with Nature as well as savoring the expectant joys that life brings. She is nurturing, grounding, and the epitome of a mother's love. Creativity and her life-giving spirit represent the seat of her powers. Her Moon goddess aspect gives her keen powers of intuition. Mawu's eyes are said to be the Moon, and that through which she can see your soul.

OFFERINGS

Caring for the Earth in honor of Mawu, even just your small patch of it, is a gift of great worth. Call your mother in her honor. Gifts born of the Earth, such as foods, crystals, water, clay, flowers, and plants, are all welcome offerings.

NINHURSAG (SUMERIAN, MESOPOTAMIAN)

Another Mother Goddess, who was believed to be the creator of all—animals, gods, and mortals—from clay, was Ninhursag, "Lady of the Mountain," also known as Nintur and Nintud, among other names. She is goddess of pregnancy and birth and midwife to the gods—protecting the child while unborn and again after birth, being the source of food for them. As with other Mother Goddesses, she also has the power of healing, which she uses to heal her true love, Enki, god of wisdom, whom (after a lapse of wisdom) she first curses for seducing their daughters and eating all the plants, then forgives and heals. She does so by absorbing his pain into her body, which results in the birth of eight new deities as gifts to humankind, earning her supreme status as giver of life and protectress from death.

Call on Ninhursag when you want to feel confident in your own powers, or when you need the time and guidance to let ideas grow and change before taking definitive action. As with all Mother Goddesses, she can be helpful in issues of fertility, in all its forms, as well as family. Let yourself connect to her to feel the power of Mother Nature and the mood-lifting benefits of engaging with her as she nourishes your soul. Seek her hand in navigating rocky ground, whether literal or emotional.

POWERS

As Mother Goddess, Ninhursag ruled over creation, with the power to give life, and the transformative power of a mother's love. She was also goddess of rocky ground, with her powers to help keep your emotions on an even keel. Her healing powers are greatest of all.

OFFERINGS

Offerings of nourishment, including wine, beer, fruits, vegetables, seeds, and nuts are appropriate on your altar when working with Ninhursag. Acts of healing and forgiveness in her name are sure signs of gratitude for her blessings as well.

OSHUN (AFRICAN)

This benevolent goddess of purity, undying love, and fertility, Oshun, is said to be the young sister of Yemaya (see page 52). She is a water orisha (goddess) in the Yoruba and Santeria religions. Legend tells us she was created to reign over the rivers and other sources of fresh water because the world lacked the loving-kindness she provided. Like other water deities, there is also a serenely seductive side to Oshun.

Renowned for her beauty, with a sweet, charming temperament to match, Oshun was constantly pursued by the gods. One day, Ogun, a warrior orisha, was in hot pursuit of Oshun. Trying to escape him, she disappeared under the river, where she was taken under the wing of Yemaya, who offered her guidance and protection. The two goddesses work as a team, with Oshun ruling over the fresh waters and Yemaya ruling over the seas, and Oshun guiding the loving, fertile, sensual aspects of relationships, while Yemaya helps bring life into the world safely, guiding the birth of the children born of these relationships.

Befitting one of the most-revered orisha in the Yoruba religion, the banks of the river bearing her name, the Osun River, in southern Nigeria, give home to a sacred forest housing all manner of shrines and sanctuaries in Oshun's honor, which is now a UNESCO World Heritage site.

Call on Oshun when life hits a barren patch, most literally for fertility related to childbirth, but also fertility related to budding romance, new ideas, new habits, new relationships in general, or new knowledge. Seek her soothing charms when stress may be preventing you from manifesting your true desires, or an even, flowing temper could help calm the choppy waters of life. In return, your faithful love of Oshun will ensure a prosperous relationship.

POWERS

Oshun has the powers to charm, seduce, and inflame love for those seeking to bear children. The great abundance of the waters she rules can bring prosperity to your life, as well as offer the soothing, healing qualities they instill and a sense of peace and happiness.

OFFERINGS

To match Oshun's sweet personality, sweet things are appropriate offerings, such as honey, oranges, cinnamon, sweet wine, and candy. Fresh water, of course, carries her spirit and can be given in offering or used in rituals or spellwork to evoke her spirit. Also, anything gold colored, the color that reflects her beauty—such as sunflowers, a favorite—will bring her great joy and contentment.

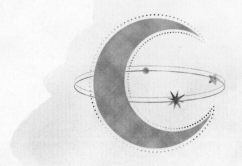

SELENE (GREEK) / LUNA (ROMAN)

The Titan goddess Selene is revered as the personification of the Moon and rules the night skies, and by association, the awe-inspiring love awakened by the fair Moon. A beautiful woman, she is often depicted wearing a crescent Moon on her head, riding her horse-drawn chariot, pulling the Moon across the skies to light them. Selene is often thought of as the Full Moon, or mother, aspect of the Triple Goddess (see page 50), along with Artemis (Waxing Moon) and Hecate (Waning Moon). She was worshipped at the New and Full Moons. She represents love, passion, and light.

Selene so loved a mortal shepherd named Endymion that she could not bear the thought of losing him. Her wish to grant him immortality was countered with perpetual youth—in sleep. Selene is said to have visited him each night as the Moon went down. Asleep, some say with his eyes open to adore his beloved, the Moon and Selene managed to create 50 daughters—the Menai, the 50 goddesses of the lunar months. Selene also had a number of children with Zeus, and others, if you believe all the accounts. Her fertility in childbearing carried over to her association with agriculture and a fertile harvest. The crystal selenite takes its name from Selene. It is a powerfully energetic stone with cleansing properties. This crystal of light can see you through dark times and lead to spiritual renewal.

Call on Selene when working to enhance your intuition, or when everyday problems or issues would benefit from a little extra light so you may see them more clearly. Her ability to bear many children lends evidence to her ability to help you bear creative fruit in any endeavor. Call on Selene when your divine goddess needs a lift—a ride in her chariot may be enough to excite your passions.

POWERS

Selene's powers are those of the Moon: healing, intuition, divine feminine energy. Her passionate charms lead to loving relationships, but not necessarily lasting ones. Her Mother Goddess tendencies rule over fertility and family issues. As traveler of the night sky, she can illuminate your journey to its safe destination.

OFFERINGS

Use Moon water to bless or cleanse your altar to Selene; anything white, silver-colored, or symbolic of the Moon will charm Selene. Moonstone and selenite are good crystals to utilize when working with Selene.

TRIPLE GODDESS

An important figure in contemporary Wicca beliefs and many other goddess-worshipping cultures, the supreme Triple Goddess, in her three forms, characterizes a female passing through life's seasonal cycle and is aligned with the Moon's mystical phases. Signifying the young maiden is the Waxing Moon; then as she grows to full adulthood and motherhood, she is represented by the Full Moon; and finally she emerges at the end of life as the wise, slightly feared, and less understood crone (the Waning Moon). Thus ends the cycle—and it signals endings—yet preparing to begin anew and reflecting the natural life cycle that all living things share. She also represents feminine energy and fierce intuitive abilities.

Each phase also has corresponding goddesses in other cultures, such as Artemis, the Greek maiden, or even the Virgin Mary, as the divine mother figure in the Catholic belief system, and Banshee (Celtic) or Spider Grandmother in Native American folklore as a crone.

The Triple Goddess is a complex philosophy, and in other cultures and ancient civilizations, she is not always represented as maiden-mother-crone in one deity, but may be a single goddess ruling over three aspects of life or society—like Brigid, goddess of fire, healing, and poetry—or a single entity comprising three goddesses—such as the Fates or the Morrigan—but she is still a powerful and revered figure.

Each Triple Goddess phase bears ample opportunity to work its energy into your goddess magic—aligning with the Moon's energetic phases adds more meaning and power to your intentions:

MAIDEN: The exhilaration of springtime and emergent opportunity; youthful beauty, confidence, spontaneity, and enthusiasm; creativity; innocence. Call on her when new beginnings and fresh starts are desired and the energies of youth can help you get there. Give gratitude for the simple joys in life.

MOTHER: The fulfillment of life—abundance; teacher, nurturer; she has stature and commands respect; call on her for issues of fertility, childbirth, and child rearing, when tough decisions need steady counsel, or when asserting yourself with authority is called for. Seek unconditional love in her arms and give gratitude by practicing self-acceptance.

CRONE: Reflects the wisdom learned of a lifetime, and a solitary stage of life, as her phase is slightly feared for its signal of death. Tap into her deep wisdom when life's mysteries present themselves, and especially for comfort and support when endings are an inevitable part of life—and not just death, but losing a job, ending a relationship, loss of a friend or dream, aging, etc. Give gratitude for the completion of a cycle and all it meant while celebrating the rebirth it makes possible.

POWERS

The Triple Goddess's powers lie in the complexity of her personality. She is at once young and confident, offers unconditional love, and can help unravel the mysteries of a lifetime. There is something to be learned from each aspect, with perhaps the opportunity for lifelong learning being her greatest power.

OFFERINGS

Make offerings to the Triple Goddess deity as one—moonstone is a powerful energy amplifier for this goddess.

For the *maiden*, consider parsley for joy and any spring flowers for beauty and freshness, as well as labradorite for its illuminating properties.

The *mother* will appreciate roses, milk, and fresh fruit, and in particular rose quartz for unconditional love.

For the *crone*, herbal offerings such as rosemary for remembrance and sage for wisdom are easy to obtain. Amethyst taps into her intuitive wisdom and clear quartz can channel any energies you can summon.

YEMAYA (AFRICAN)

This benevolent Mother Goddess and water spirit has roots in Nigeria, in western Africa, where she is revered by the Yoruba faith as the mother of all orishas, or gods and goddesses, of the Yoruba pantheon. Yemaya is worshipped as orisha, goddess, of the oceans and source of all waters, especially the western African river Ogun—and thus, life Her influence also extends to Cuba and Brazil, where she also rules as ocean goddess. Yemaya is a women of mystery, and her energy and secrets run as deep as the oceans she tends. And as with Marie Laveau (see page 66), her worship and traditions were introduced to America by the enslaved Africans brought to the country as early as the sixteenth century.

Yemaya, whose name means "mother whose children are fish," is frequently shown as a beautiful mermaid, and her watery nature is tied to the Moon and all things with feminine mystique. This maternal goddess rules over all that pertains to women, especially pregnancy and childbirth. It is told that, upon her water breaking, great floods burst forth carrying the first humans born of her. As we are all born of water, we are all connected to Yemaya and can see and experience her spirit in others.

In addition to the important work she does for mothers, she also guards and protects all those who live, work, travel, or play on the water.

Her gentle, flowing nature soothes, calms, and instills confidence, and her generosity is as boundless as the seas she rules. She calls us to her shores as a mother's open arms beckon with the promise of safety and acceptance. But like all waters, when her forces are angered and tested, she can be destructive to those who threaten.

Yemaya's spirit is said to be summoned with a gourd rattle or conch shell, which is said to contain her voice. (Hold one to your ear: Can you hear her whisper?) Call on Yemaya's graceful spirit for any issues regarding fertility, pregnancy, and motherhood—even marriage—and on her quiet strength to fight anything that threatens harm. Issues of need, whether monetary, love, friendship, or security, are filled easily by her.

POWERS

The force of Yemaya's nurturing powers can be felt most strongly when near a body of water, but she is available to you anytime, just by incorporating a water element—even the sounds of rain or the ocean surf—into your spellwork. A connection with Yemaya can help ease suffering, cultivate self-love, increase fertility, and provide security in all aspects of life. Her love brings hope to all who experience it and fosters a sense of harmony and peace.

OFFERINGS

There is no paucity of appropriate offerings to Yemaya. Traditional offerings include anything to do with the sea or rivers, such as seashells, river stones, or blue beads and crystals representing water; also clean water; cocoa, coconut, corn, jewelry, molasses, peanuts, perfume, and white flowers; and offerings made in quantities of seven, for the seven seas.

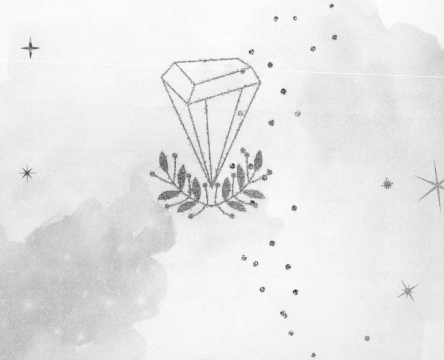

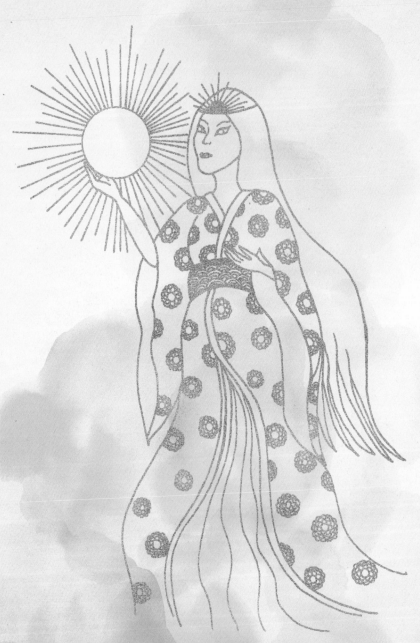

Amaterasu, Japanese goddess of the sun

Goddesses of Relationships, Truth, and Forgiveness

Healthy relationships require a strong degree of compassion, a steady dose of truth, and a deep well of forgiveness. The goddesses here can help with all your needs for developing and maintaining successful relationships. They have suffered as we all do, then chosen forgiveness and healing to move forward. Their wisdom is peace and power, and their song is harmony.

The concept of forgiveness wasn't always as common as it is today. It was frequently believed that Fate would determine one's destiny, based on good deeds or bad. When forgiveness enters the mix, either of one's self or others, it is a powerful ally in improving relationships.

Real friendships are like gold. Work with these goddesses to tend to yours and seek their companionship if loss or loneliness troubles you. Be open to receiving the light and joy of their messages and listen carefully for their words of forgiveness. Invite them for a chat and offer a toast with the nectar of the gods they pour. With them, there is no pressure for performance, just the honest ease of compassion and companionship. Savor the friendships and learn from each other's experiences.

CELEBRATE THE GODDESS

Rejoice in your newfound friendships and celebrate the goddess. Honor her special days, work with her symbols, or just appreciate her point of view more with these tips and facts.

Amaterasu (Japanese), page 59

This Sun goddess's return to the skies is celebrated on December 21, winter solstice. Mirrors are sacred to Amaterasu. Clean all the mirrors in your home and let the true beauty of your surroundings shine, including your reflection.

Clementia (Roman) / Eleos (Greek), page 61

An olive branch, and the significance of its symbolism of forgiveness and peace, is sacred to Clementia. Find the best-quality olive oil you can afford and use it to season your food in her honor.

Iris (Greek), page 62

Iris, messenger of the gods, has a message for you: Contact all those friends and family you've been too busy to acknowledge lately and nurture those relationships that sustain you in difficult times.

Kuan Yin (Chinese), page 63

The nineteenth day of the second lunar month honors Kuan Yin's birthday, but this beloved goddess of compassion is available to you 24/7. Add a chime of compassion to your altar and begin each day reciting her mantra: *Om mani padme hum,* which invokes her blessings.

Ma'at (Egyptian), page 65

This widely revered goddess was typically celebrated with offerings of food, wine, and incense. Light your favorite scented candle at dinner tonight and set a place at the table for Ma'at.

Marie Laveau (American), page 66

Marking three Xs on her crypt is a traditional (though illegal) ritual when asking for favors from this Voodoo Queen, or acknowledging those granted; you may simply want to do so in your journal or grimoire as you set intentions and assess outcomes.

Rhiannon (Welsh), page 68

March 4 is the day designated to celebrate Rhiannon. As she is particularly associated with songbirds, feed the birds as a way to honor her, or just take a walk in nature and see how many different birdsongs you recognize.

Veritas (Roman) / Aletheia (Greek), page 70

Veritas held supreme reign in Roman society, as truthfulness was a quality deemed most important of all. Have a little fun with Veritas, playing two truths and a lie with some friends.

White Buffalo Calf Woman (Native American), page 71

This goddess brought her People the Seven Sacred Ceremonies to live a good life. For the next week, do something kind for another each day, honor the Earth, or teach a child what it means to be generous.

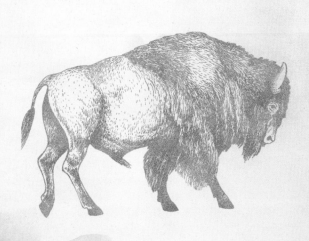

As goddess rides across the sky, as Sun, or Moon,
or rainbow high, so signaled here on Earth am I:

To open ears and mind and eyes
to notice what the heart doth spy;

to hear a loved one's precious sigh
or dream of that which beckons nigh.

To see what's right before my eyes,
to choose the truth above a lie.

To seek forgiveness, just and true,
and offer it in kind to you.

O goddess, draw this precious veil,
that worlds unknown revealed do hail.

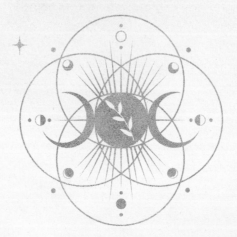

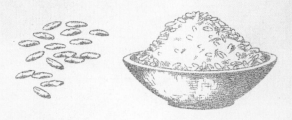

AMATERASU (JAPANESE)

Sun goddess Amaterasu—supreme deity of the Shinto religion—whose
name means "illuminating heaven," is goddess of unity, sustenance,
and protection. She is a kind, benevolent goddess credited with
creating rice to feed her people and teaching the craft of raising
silkworms and weaving their threads into fabric, which she made into
robes for the gods.

As little brothers are wont to do, hers—Susanoo, god of chaos—
among other things, desecrated her palace and destroyed her rice
paddies. Distraught at the violence and destruction, Amaterasu fled
to a cave for safety, refusing to come out. The world was thrown into
utter darkness and, the longer she stayed, the grimmer things became.
With no light, there grew no food. People were starving and the Earth
was cold. No pleading could change her mind, until Uzume, goddess of
joy, began an unusual and joyous dance, which turned into a striptease
resulting in bawdy laughter and celebration outside the cave. Tempted
by the noise, Amaterasu peeked out from the cave and was met by her
reflection in a mirror planted there. So taken was she by her never-
before-seen beauty, she was distracted long enough to be pulled from
the cave and the door closed fast behind her to prevent re-entry. The
people rejoiced as the Sun returned to the sky, dispelling winter, and life
returned to normal.

Seek Amaterasu's counsel in all things friendship and unity, when in search of blessings and harmony, for advice as guardian of your family, inspiration for beauty, and when a return of healing and joy after darkness is needed.

POWERS

As goddess of the Sun, Amaterasu literally shines light on everything, bringing life, clarity, vision, nourishment, and order to the world. She has the power to unite us in kinship and vision, bringing peace and harmony to our world.

OFFERINGS

Mirrors and other reflective objects, chrysanthemums, jewels, rice, silk, and yellow (like the Sun) candles and other objects, such as clothing or altar coverings, are appropriate and appreciated offerings to Amaterasu.

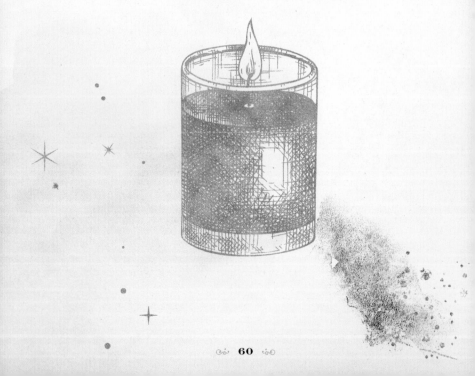

CLEMENTIA (ROMAN) / ELEOS (GREEK)

Clementia personifies mercy. Her name means "gentleness," especially in association with punishment. She is often depicted with either a scepter and an offering dish, or holding an olive or laurel branch, which signifies both victory and its ensuing peace. Her worship began when she was given goddess status as the virtue of Julius Caesar (though not all agreed he was so virtuous).

Call on Clementia when feelings of hurt or anger blind your compassion to others, or when a little self-compassion is in order.

POWERS

Kind and compassionate, Clementia gives comfort to all who seek it from her. Forgiveness and mercy are also powers Clementia bestows on her worshippers, which can help you walk in another's shoes before passing judgment.

OFFERINGS

Coins, olive oil, laurel leaves or bay leaves, and a kind word are offerings Clementia will gladly accept. Using bay leaves in cooking will infuse your foods with nourishing mercy and forgiveness.

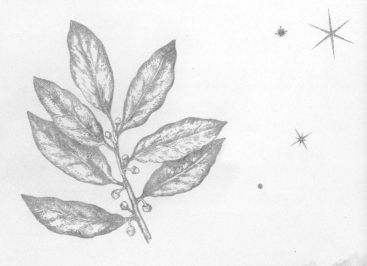

IRIS (GREEK)

Depicted as a beautiful, winged goddess, Iris—goddess of the rainbow—is the daughter of Electra (best known for killing her mother, Queen Clytemnestra, to avenge the death of her father, King Agamemnon), messenger to the gods, and loyal servant to Hera (see page 41). Iris poured nectar for the gods from her pitcher and carried their messages from Mount Olympus to Earth and the Underworld—where she also retrieved water from the River Styx, which was used in solemn oath-taking ceremonies of the gods. Should you choose to lie under oath, the water would leave you speechless. Her symbol, the rainbow, reflects the connection between the heavens and Earth. Iris is also associated with water. She is the soothing stillness after the storm and the calming words of mediation.

Call on Iris when your head and your heart are not in harmony; she will help you trust your intuition. She is equally as powerful when you need to speak clearly so your message is heard and understood. When working with this goddess, seek help eliminating negative self-talk and letting go of people, circumstances, behaviors, and things that no longer serve you. Evoke her when clear and healing communication is needed as a bridge to kindness and understanding.

POWERS

Comfortable in the realms of gods as well as mortals, Iris can help keep the peace and make sure everyone stays on the same page. Her role as servant to others breeds the power to be flexible in all situations to ensure a positive outcome. This goddess shines brightly in matters of communication, faithfulness, and duty, but can neglect self-care while tending to the needs of others.

OFFERINGS

Tempt Iris with crystals or prisms that will catch the light and break it into the colors of the rainbow. Flowers are a favorite, especially the iris. Anything water related also makes a soothing offering.

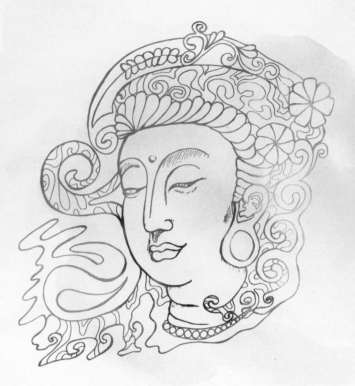

KUAN YIN (CHINESE)

The beautiful Kuan Yin is the revered Chinese goddess of mercy,
compassion, kindness, and love. Though she originated in China, her
influence spread far and wide. She is often depicted in flowing white
robes with a water jar, holding the life-giving liquid, and a willow branch,
with which she blesses the world with peace. When she is seated upon
a pink lotus, the message is peace and harmony. Her story of having
been blessed with 1,000 arms, each with an eye in the palm, tells us of
her compassion for all of human suffering, as she sees all in need and
reaches out to tend to them. One legend holds that, upon being killed
by her father's decree for refusing to marry as he wished (for which she
forgave her executioner), then transported to hell, she played music as
flowers bloomed all around, transforming it into a paradise.

Call on Kuan Yin to fill your reservoir of compassion when you're feeling a bit tapped out. She also blesses with the wisdom of adaptability and compromise if your relationships are feeling a bit one-sided, and instills the ability to forgive in the most difficult times, as the forgiveness is really our salvation. When your "hell" needs a little more paradise, seek Kuan Yin's help.

POWERS

Kuan Yin can help rescue you from any harm set to befall you—just call her name with belief. The *Lotus Sutra* tells us of ten specific protections Kuan Yin may be petitioned to grant—from fire, water, falling, politics, prison, curses, demons, evil beasts, disputes, and of children—by bestowing good fortune.

OFFERINGS

Kuan Yin actually requires no offerings in her name. If gifts to her in gratitude will make you feel better, consider lotus flowers, oolong tea leaves, orange, pomegranate, and willow branches. The greatest gift to her is an act of aid or compassion to others in need.

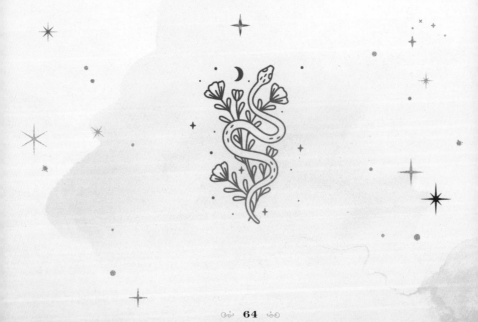

MA'AT (EGYPTIAN)

Egyptian goddess of harmony, justice, truth, and universal order, Ma'at,
daughter of Sun god Ra, was born from the chaos with which Ra created
the world. She was supremely important in her time, serving as keeper
of world order and choreographer of the celestial dance of the Sun,
Moon, and stars. She was frequently shown wearing an ostrich feather
on her head—her feather of truth—with which your heart was compared
upon death as a measure of one's good worth. During the Weighing
of the Heart of the Soul, if, on the Scales of Justice, one's heart weight
balanced the feather, you were judged to be without burden and granted
permission to proceed to the Afterlife; if it was heavier, your journey was
over. And so Egyptians lived their lives accordingly.

Ma'at represented the perfect Egyptian woman, and was the spirit
of creation and your conscience: To live in harmony with her spirit, to
care for others as well as Earth, was to live a good life.

Call on Ma'at to help restore balance when your world feels like it's
spinning out of control and the truth can help to re-establish order.

POWERS

Ma'at had the power to decide whose life on Earth was not the end of the
journey and whose ended at death. Her influence ensured the truth was
spoken and her guiding principles provided the structure for a peaceful,
harmonious existence.

OFFERINGS

Sacred to Ma'at are feathers, aloe, frankincense, orris root (often an
ingredient in potpourri, which could stand in, if needed), and roses. Also
any gift or offering you wish to make to any other goddess you work
with is appropriate for Ma'at.

MARIE LAVEAU (AMERICAN)

The history of Marie Laveau, perhaps the most influential American practitioner of the magical arts and Voodoo Queen of New Orleans, is largely one of oral tradition. Born in 1801 (the exact date is disputed; some say 1794) in New Orleans, Louisiana—the illegitimate daughter of a wealthy Creole plantation owner (white) and his mistress (African and American Indian)—she is said to have been both bewitchingly beautiful and descended from a powerful Saint-Domingue (Haiti) priestess.

Raised Catholic, a religion she never abandoned, Marie had an interest in African religious traditions that arose from her mother's beliefs. The mystical religion of Voodoo, based in African spiritual beliefs, was brought to New Orleans during the period of the transatlantic slave trade, where it grew in tradition and numbers supported by a wave of immigrants following the Saint-Domingue (Haiti) Revolution, and flourished there in the eighteenth century. It was shortly after this period that Marie honed her skills under the tutelage of a Voodoo doctor in New Orleans.

Following the death (some say disappearance!) of Marie's first husband (leaving her with two children to raise), she worked as a hairdresser and sometimes nurse. Perhaps owing to her compassionate nature and keen ability to listen, her clients—wealthy and not, Creole and not—regarded Marie as a confidante, spilling family secrets, drama, intel, dreams and desires, business issues, and problems and gossip of all kinds during their time in her chair. Thus was born Marie's introduction to the community as the great Voodoo Queen as she counseled, charmed, blessed, and foretold of good fortunes (relying heavily on information she learned about such!). Her second marriage saw the birth of several more children, which required her to quit hairdressing to manage her household—and gave her more time to consult with her clients. Her reputation and power were growing, too. And although Marie was revered for her helpful magic, tales abounded of the outcomes of those who offended her, producing great fear mixed with reverence for her power.

Marie reigned as New Orleans' Voodoo Queen from about 1830 to about 1850, during which time she was leader of all public Voodoo events, as well as private and secret gatherings, regularly conducting rituals and ceremonies where it was described that people became "possessed" (with lots of music, singing, and dancing, believed to help one connect with the spirit world), which generated much gossip, as well as publicity—and income, as she began charging for admission!

Staying active well into her seventies, using her power to serve her community, Marie died in 1881 and is reputed to be buried in St. Louis Cemetery No. 1, where her grave attracts worshippers and the curious alike, and where traditional offerings are left in hopes of her spirit still granting favors in this life.

Invoke Marie's name, as is traditional, when casting any spells for love (and casting dice, they say!). Call on her healing spirit to ease stress or illness, her strength for protection, and her wisdom in navigating interpersonal relationships with ease, charity, and compassion.

POWERS

Marie Laveau was hailed for her powers of nursing and healing the sick. Her generosity to the poor and those in need and her compassion to her community were widely known. Her wisdom, counsel, and prophecy were widely sought for matters of the heart and other personal concerns—from good luck to fertility to politics, wealth, and exorcisms. Marie dispensed charms and potions for all manner of healing and protection (using remnants of her Catholic beliefs to inspire such), for which her wealthy white clients paid handsomely.

OFFERINGS

Traditional offerings of food, coins, Mardi Gras beads, rum, flowers, and candles are said to call forth Marie's spirit to grant favors and wishes requested.

RHIANNON (WELSH)

Horse goddess and goddess of magic—as well as goddess of the Moon—Rhiannon seems an unlikely goddess for this category, but she is also goddess of true love and domestic bliss, and there is much to learn from her. Rhiannon married Pwyll, Prince of Dyfed, who fell in love with her at first sight as she rode past on her beautiful white horse. Accompanying her were three songbirds with the most beautiful songs—said to wake the dead or gently lull one to sleep! They had a son, Pryderi, who vanished mysteriously shortly after birth. The nursemaids on watch, to avoid trouble themselves, falsely accused Rhiannon of killing her newborn. Trouble ensued, as did an unusual sentence for Rhiannon: seven years sitting outside the castle walls to tell her tale to anyone who had not heard—then carrying them to court on her back like a horse! She bore her fate with dignity, if not sadness, and her husband stood by her side.

Meanwhile, her infant son mysteriously appeared in a barn, was adopted by the couple who found him, and grew into a talented equestrian with seemingly magical powers. His adopted father began to suspect who he was, and so returned him to his mother. Rhiannon, thus exonerated, returned to her roles as wife, mother, and princess. From her, we learn to face what life gives us the best way we can and without blame, that the truth triumphs, all things are possible with time, and loyalty and love in relationships can sustain us through dark times until the light returns.

Call on Rhiannon for matters of domestic happiness, when patience seems elusive, and strength beyond your means is needed to reach your goals. She can be an ally in your Moon magic work, if you so desire.

POWERS

Rhiannon demonstrates great strength—physical, spiritual, and mental—in the face of significant challenges and the patience of a saint in awaiting the redemption of truth. Her beauty and powers of courage are great sources of inspiration. She has the power to reveal truth in dreams.

OFFERINGS

Anything related to horses or birds will delight Rhiannon. Consider also safely burning white candles, or place white flowers in a vase, a moonstone, or a gift on your altar in gratitude to the people in your life who sustain you.

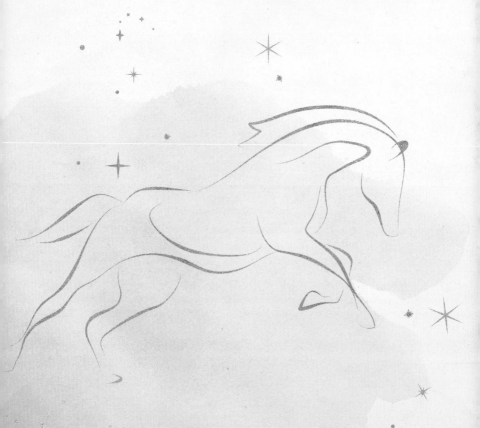

VERITAS (ROMAN) / ALETHEIA (GREEK)

Veritas was goddess of truth and sincerity. Her name means "truth" and her Greek counterpart's name, Aletheia, equates to "that which is obvious," or not hidden. It is the very essence of something that exists for its own beauty and purpose, not to be obscured or left unacknowledged. She is the daughter of Zeus (or Saturn, or created by Prometheus, depending on which story you read) and mother of Virtue. Known to be an elusive goddess, Veritas frequently could be found hiding in a well—but only if you were determined to track her down. She is often pictured dressed in white, or fully nude and holding a hand mirror to reflect the "naked truth."

Look first within yourself to recognize your truth before calling on Veritas to help you live it.

POWERS
The power of Veritas is revealed in the understanding of the power of truth: to heal, to set you free, to honor your ideals and purpose. Her powers of courage bolster the will to pursue truth and speak it at all times. Though truth may be difficult to find sometimes, persistence is key and the reward is great.

OFFERINGS
Anything reflective, like a mirror, or more personally reflective, like journaling, with Veritas is a meaningful offering. In addition, bittersweet or white chrysanthemum for truth, fern for sincerity, or mint for virtue make lovely gifts on your altar.

WHITE BUFFALO CALF WOMAN
(NATIVE AMERICAN)

The White Buffalo Calf Woman, a legend of the Lakota People as well as other Native American tribes, is known as the messenger from ancestors departed and as a healer. She is also a teacher and peacemaker. White Buffalo Calf Woman first appeared to two Native American warriors out hunting food for their People. On sighting her, they were faced with a large white buffalo, but as she drew closer, she transformed into a beautiful Indian maiden who foretold of bringing their People the Sacred Pipe and its secrets. She dissolved one warrior for his bad behavior toward her and instructed the other to go tell his People to await her arrival.

As promised, she appeared some days later to deliver the Sacred Pipe, which she taught them to use in seven sacred prayer rituals for purification, child naming, healing, making relatives, marriage, vision quest, and the sun dance. Using these tools guaranteed care of the land and survival of the Nation. When her mission was complete, she left in the same way she came—promising to return someday to, once again, bring harmony to the world, signaled by the birth of the white buffalo calf.

Call on White Buffalo Calf Woman when your world, or the world at large, can be healed by peace, harmony, and understanding. Invoke White Buffalo Calf Woman when your concern is for our planet and healing Earth.

POWERS

White Buffalo Calf Woman brings peace and harmony to all those who honor her and, with those gifts, hope in times of trouble. She teaches us to walk and work together for the good of all and to honor the lessons of your ancestors in your actions today. Her powers of respect, humility, and wisdom help us tame the chaos and live as one.

OFFERINGS

Feathers, dried herbs, especially sage, and tobacco, and fresh water are traditional offerings. When working on behalf of the world and its health and environment, White Buffalo Calf Woman sends blessings from above.

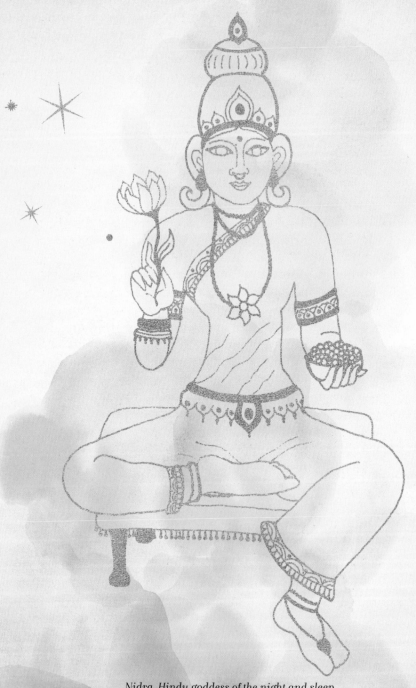

Nidra, Hindu goddess of the night and sleep

Goddesses of the Home, Hearth, and Healing

Your home is your sanctuary—your sacred place of love and nurture, comfort, safety, discovery, and healing.

The goddesses who reside here are selfless; their talents are many and their work is never done. They work from morning to night tending to everyone's needs to be sure the home is a secure, welcoming, safe, and happy place. They'll even tuck you into sweet dreams when you ask.

These goddesses of domestic bliss can inspire, heal, soothe, and restore. They are kind, loving, wise, creative, protective, forgiving, and fiery!

Working with these goddesses puts you in charge of all that happens within your home. They can help protect your home's inhabitants from evil, banish negative energies, keep the peace, set intentions to transform your life, and simply reflect all you have to be grateful for. They can also teach the value of self-care when days are spent thinking about and caring for others' needs and wants. Their goal is to help create a place to thrive in whatever ways you wish.

CELEBRATE THE GODDESS

Rejoice in your newfound friendships and celebrate the goddess. Honor her special days, work with her symbols, or just better appreciate her point of view with these tips and facts.

Airmid (Celtic), page 77

Legend says 365 herbs grew where Airmid's slain brother was buried—one for each of his joints and sinews. In her spirit, plant your favorite herb and talk to it to gain its healing wisdom. Celebrate the "weeds" pushing through the sidewalk: they have something to teach us, too.

Bao Gu (Chinese), page 78

Celebrate this goddess of healing by scheduling all those preventive appointments you've been putting off: Mammogram? Check. Dental cleaning? Check. Other? Check. Or, try acupuncture for what ails.

Brigid (Celtic), page 79

Imbolc, February 2, is the day honoring Brigid, and is a celebration of the Earth's reawakening. Light candles and turn on all the lights in your home to banish the darkness. Celebrate sunrise, the time of Brigid's birth, and its sacred flame of new opportunities.

Caer Ibormeith (Celtic), page 81

This fairy/goddess is feted on Samhain, October 31, the day each year she transforms from swan to human or vice versa. Recreate the peaceful lake where she lives by placing a birdbath in your garden and inviting fairies in to take a dip.

Cerridwen (Celtic), page 82

July 3 celebrates Cerridwen. Put your largest cooking cauldron to work transforming raw ingredients into a feast to nourish friends and family. Honor her Triple Goddess aspect by celebrating all the women in your life through all their ages and appreciate each for her strengths.

Epione (Greek), page 84

To celebrate Epione, goddess of soothing pain, enjoy a soothing ritual to ease the day: mani-pedi, mini facial, time in meditation, listen to favorite music, take a walk, soak in a hot tub . . .

Frigg (Norse), page 85

Winter solstice, generally December 21, marks the time to honor Frigg. In thanks to Odin for restoring their son, Baldur, to life after being killed by an arrow made of mistletoe, Frigg declared the mistletoe a plant of love. Have a kiss under the mistletoe in her honor.

Gabija (Lithuanian), page 87

Goddess of the hearth fire, traditionally fed with bread and salt—bake some bread, or do whatever feeds your inner fire to keep it glowing.

Hestia (Greek) / Vesta (Roman), page 88

June 9 is the festival Vestalia, honoring hearth goddess Vesta. To celebrate both goddesses of the hearth, have a campfire, gather friends and family, and celebrate the sacred hearth and its fire in uniting family.

Nidra (Hindu), page 90

This goddess of sleep knows the power of beauty sleep. Take a nap; create a bedtime ritual to relax you, and ease into dreamland; keep a journal of your dreams and look for patterns—they may be messages from Nidra.

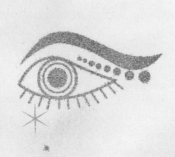

Goddess, please do share your spell
to dampen swift each fire that swells.

So, buoyed I be by your great charms
that never will my home know harm,

Just joy and bounty far and wide—
each reaped with gratitude and pride.

This home and hearth, dear goddess, bless,
that love and time reveal our best.

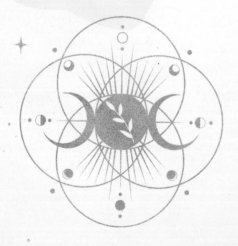

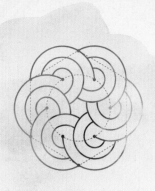

AIRMID (CELTIC)

This Irish goddess of healing hails from the ancient magical race of the Tuatha Dé Danann. The story is told that her tears of grief, wept over her brother's grave, gave birth to a garden of healing herbs—so vast in scope it was believed to represent the complete array of available herbs. With wondrous curiosity, Airmid gathered the herbs in her cloak and worked with them, as they revealed their secrets to her.

She became keeper of all wisdom and knowledge of herbal healing magic and was particularly skilled at healing soldiers injured in battle.

Whether your battles are more of the modern-day kind, or just tussles with family, or a wish to use Nature's medicine to heal in general, speak to Airmid. She will listen.

POWERS

Airmid's powers are of magic, patience, growth, healing, the creation of healing waters, and her vast herbal knowledge, which she will generously share with those who ask and respect the knowledge, using it only for good. Evoke Airmid while gardening; she will imbue your plants with her magical powers to bolster their natural healing abilities.

OFFERINGS

Place any single herb or variety of dried herbs in a mortar with a pestle and place it on your altar in Airmid's honor. Add a vase of fresh herbs or herbal tea for the wondrous power of aroma to heal. Celebrate Airmid during the Waxing Moon to promote healing. Grow aloe vera or chamomile for Airmid to bless, so the plants' powers to comfort and heal will aid you when needed.

BAO GU (CHINESE)

Bao Gu was a Chinese woman and physician, living in fourth-century China. For her extraordinary kindness and healing skills, she was given goddess status—of healing and medicine, especially using traditional Chinese medicine techniques, including acupuncture and the natural healing powers of herbs. She learned magic and medicine while being raised in a monastery, later marrying another respected physician and scholar, an apprentice of her father. Her learning, skills, and experience were duly noted at the time, as they were far outside the typical woman's role. In addition to the herbal research she did, she was quite interested in the healing powers of water.

Call on Bao Gu when your relationships could use a prescription of a little TLC, or when her herbalist skills can combine with aromatherapy for a little healing self-care.

POWERS

Bao Gu was a leader before her time. Her powers were her gifts of courage, healing, and compassion, and her service to her people. She also possessed the gifts of magic, curiosity, creativity, and great learning. With these gifts, she brought great healing to the world and left a legacy of knowledge with which to carry on her traditions.

OFFERINGS

Try a spa bath at home in honor of Bao Gu, using Himalayan salt to ease aches and pains and nourish the skin. Other appropriate offerings are clean water, fresh herbs, and respect for the power of a single woman to make a difference in the lives of many.

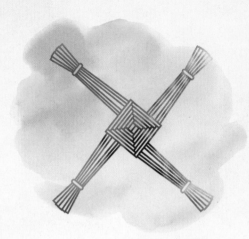

BRIGID (CELTIC)

Another goddess of the Tuatha Dé Danann, Brigid, whose name means "exalted one," was goddess of the hearth, and, among other duties, patron of the sacred household fires, which warmed the family and provided the fuel for the magic of cooking the meals. As such, her symbol is the cauldron. Tradition held that the woman of the house, while performing the daily chore of putting the fire to bed for the evening, pleaded with Brigid for protection of all who dwelt within. Brigid also represents the fires of creativity and in this role is much revered as the goddess of poets, and her sacred wells are visited for the healing power of their waters.

Tales are told of St. Brigid weaving a cross from rushes as she calmed the restless soul of a chieftain who lay dying. Hanging a replica of St. Brigid's cross on your front door or entryway, especially on Imbolc (see page 74), is thought to protect from evil spirits and fire, and ward off hunger in the home.

Call on Brigid when her warming fires of inner healing can help you take on the duty of caring for home and family. Seek her warmth to restore your energy. Be inspired by her poetry to lend a little magic to your words.

POWERS

Brigid's powers are born of the eternal flame she tends, which nurtures and cares for the home, ignites our powers of creativity, sparks the imagination, burns brightly in our hearts as passion, transforms, and melts winter into the rebirth of spring, illuminating our hope. Her eternal flame is the light by which we find our way.

OFFERINGS

A crackling fire lit in Brigid's honor gives you a place to sit with her in quiet conversation. Listen carefully—the crackle is Brigid speaking to you. No fireplace? Open the windows and let the Sun shine in, along with the breeze bearing Brigid's wisdom, or place some twigs on your altar representing the fuel for her fires. Offerings of food and wine are traditional ways to acknowledge Brigid, especially when leftover from a family meal. Place a cauldron on your altar in which to light a candle when working with Brigid. Write a poem in her honor.

CAER IBORMEITH (CELTIC)

Goddess of dreams and prophecy, Caer Ibormeith, daughter of a fairy king, is descended from the legendary Tuatha Dé Danann. Caer was a beautiful, independent, shape-shifting goddess who lived her life alternating one year as a woman and one year as a swan—morphing every year on Samhain. She chose her true love by appearing to him in his dreams for a year, singing songs of love, only to disappear when he reached for her, which left him so lovesick he was unable to eat. For three years, first by his mother, then his father, and finally a local king, the search for this unknown beauty ensued. Finally, she was located—but in the guise of a swan among 150 others, all linked by a silver chain. He had to identify her and call to her for them to be united. He did—she was the most beautiful; they were—he, too, became a swan (temporarily); and the enchanting love song they sang as they flew off together cast a sleep spell of three days over all those who were near. As swans mate for life, this union has a happy ending.

Work with Caer Ibormeith when prophetic dreams can bring you the guidance you need to meet your goals on your terms, when sleep eludes, and when intuition needs a boost of clarity.

POWERS

Caer's real powers lie in her independence and her ability to love unconditionally yet without giving up who she is. She's also blessed with musical talent to soothe and delight. It can bring on blissful sleep and peaceful dreams.

OFFERINGS

Swan images on your altar, silver, music, clean water, and white candles are all offerings that Caer Ibormeith will gladly accept. A short meditation on your gratitude for her gift of a good night's rest, right before bed, can be effective, too.

CERRIDWEN (CELTIC)

Cerridwen, also known as the White Goddess and Crone, was a multifaceted goddess and one of the most powerful witches in Celtic mythology, embodying all three aspects of the Triple Goddess: maiden, mother, and crone. Among the many realms she ruled over were the Moon, magic, Nature, creation, and astrology. She also tended her great cauldron, in which her herbal potions transformed into potent potables that delivered beauty, imparted wisdom, and nourished inspiration. As such, her cauldron is also symbolic of transformation and rebirth.

Though the crone aspect of Cerridwen reveals her darker side and its search for justice based on wisdom earned, she was also a life-giving mother figure, especially devoted to her children, particularly her less-than-beautiful son, Morfran, whom she was dedicated to helping succeed in life. With a magic elixir created just for Morfran, to transform him into a brilliant and handsome man with the gift of knowledge of the future, things did not go exactly as she planned, but they worked out well in the end. In the process, she used her shape-shifting skills to adapt to the changing circumstances until success was had.

In whatever way you need her, call on Cerridwen to help nourish you when you're feeling depleted. Cerridwen is also a key to navigating change and transformation in life—especially on the fly. Evoke her energies to embrace that change and gracefully move on to the next phase of your life. She can also give you a boost when you're stuck in an unproductive routine.

POWERS

Cerridwen is a powerful, resourceful witch who offers divine inspiration, unending love, and the prophecy of change. Her magical cauldron, which she continually tends, symbolizes transformation: the transformation achieved with knowledge and power, of heat applied to food to cook it and nourish the body, as a symbol of birth and rebirth transforming lives, and the place where her potent potions are created, which can bless or take away life—and where wisdom sprinkled with inspiration uplifts her followers. Her unique gifts have earned her status as the goddess of witches and wizards.

OFFERINGS

Place any combination of six herbs in a cauldron on your altar in honor of the elixir made for her son. Decorate with fresh white flowers anywhere you want to receive Cerridwen. Leave offerings representing the four elements of air, fire, earth, and water. If you're a baker, consider creating a sourdough starter, in a representative cauldron, as Cerridwen was also associated with grain. When the starter is well tended, its replenishing qualities of mimic her bottomless cauldron—and your baking wisdom and inspiration that can be shared with friends.

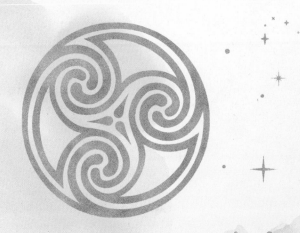

EPIONE (GREEK)

Goddess of soothing pain, Epione was the wife of Asclepius, Greek god of medicine, and mother of the five Asclepiades, or goddesses of health and healing: Aegle, goddess of radiant good health, Aceso, goddess of curing illness; Hygieia, goddess of cleanliness, disease prevention, and long life; Iaso, goddess of healing and recovery; and Panacea, goddess of cure-alls, or the cure itself.

Call on Epione to help soothe pain in all its forms. Her presence can be the balm needed to bring calm and usher in true healing.

POWERS

Though not much is known about Epione, her legacy of soothing is infamous and the power of healing is the mission of her family.

OFFERINGS

These selfless goddesses, and the god Asclepius, value gratitude and acts of kindness above all. But an altar dedicated to them is a powerful presence in a home, and simple offerings of salt and clean water for cleansing, as well as fresh herbs for healing, will help draw their powers to you.

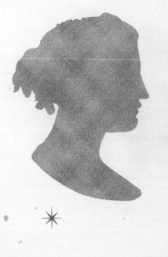

FRIGG (NORSE)

Associated with domesticity and all it affords—love, marriage, companionship, motherhood, and nurturing, Frigg—Norse goddess extraordinaire, Queen of Asgard, and wife of Odin, all-father and most powerful Norse god—is the chief domestic officer. In her powerful position as Odin's wife, she is an equal partner, granted the right to sit on the high throne with him, where she has a magnificent view of the world. Here, amplified by her practice of Norse magic (*seidr*), she can see far into the future, yet, wisely, she does not reveal all she sees. Her significant duties include being goddess of marriage, childbirth, motherhood, wisdom, and weaving. As an expert weaver, she is said to have woven the clouds, as well as the fates of all, including the untimely death of a son, Baldor, whose fate she could not undo despite her best efforts. To protect her son, she pleaded with every plant and animal on Earth to do him no harm—all agreed, except the mistletoe. Unfortunately, Loki, a trickster god, resented Frigg and so made a dart of mistletoe and threw it at Baldor. It pierced his heart and killed him. Unable to secure his release from the Queen of the Dead, Frigg is sometimes sought for her comfort on the loss of a loved one.

Her name means "beloved," and she signifies all things domestic tranquility. Friday, named for Frigg, is thus designated the best day for a wedding!

Seek her wisdom in matters of hearth and home and invite her in any time your goddess energies are running low. Call on Frigg to restore a balance of power when things seem to be out of sync, or skills of diplomacy are needed to reach agreement. Devotees also sought help regarding domestic crafts and cottage industries. If you have a home-based business or are sole proprietor of a business, put Frigg on your board.

POWERS

Frigg's powers were most closely aligned with matters of marriage and all things home and family. She is also an independent woman, able to be partner, mother, friend, and wife while keeping her own identity fully intact. She is extremely clever and uses this power to her advantage. She also had the power to foretell the future, blessed with the wisdom to keep her secrets—though she was believed to be weaver of the fates as a result.

OFFERINGS

Keep your altar to Frigg clean and tidy and place upon it offerings of wine or wool. Spend some time volunteering to help other women; make peace in your family where it's needed; retake your marriage vows. Clean your house!

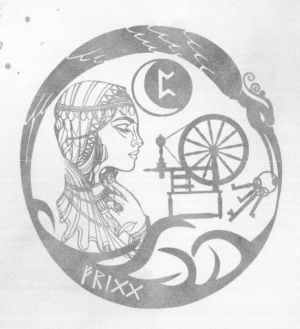

GABIJA (LITHUANIAN)

Goddess of the home fires and guardian of the home and family, like the Greek goddess Hestia (page 88), Gabija is charged with tending the flame that is the center of the home. Unlike Hestia, though, she is more aggressive—fiery!—in spirit and must be tended to accordingly. When she is put to bed each night, her ashes are neatly swept to smolder through the night; she is given a bowl of fresh water with which to bathe and kindly asked to stay put. While Gabija intends no harm—she provides the means for warmth and nourishment, after all—she is a bit high maintenance. Treat her with respect at all times.

In Lithuanian tradition, a new bride is given fire from her mother's hearth to ignite her own home fires, ensuring an auspicious start to her new married life.

Call on Gabija for protection of the home and family, especially from thieves and evil forces. Seek her light at new beginnings or when darkness temporarily obscures your intuition. Savor her message of daily rest and renewal with self-care to keep your fires burning so you can lovingly care for your family.

POWERS
Gabija commands respect due to her potential destructive nature, but rewards warmly when treated with care. She provides the fuel to transform food into nourishment for the family and light to see clearly when darkness threatens.

OFFERINGS
Food, especially bread, and salt are traditional offerings for Gabija, placed respectfully by the fire. Red objects, whether food, candles, crystals, or others, are also appropriate.

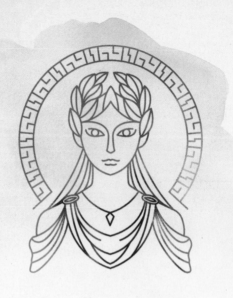

HESTIA (GREEK) / VESTA (ROMAN)

The Greek goddess Hestia was a virgin goddess dedicated to the hearth, home, family, and community. The original domestic goddess, this kind and forgiving figure was widely worshipped and held sacred in the home, where she tended the unending hearth fires—to warm, nourish, and sustain. The hearth, symbolizing the soul of a home (much as today's kitchen), was a gathering place for family life, not just meals, and so sacrifices to Hestia there were common. Offerings of wine and food in her honor were typical, with toasts beginning and ending with "To Hestia!" Relinquishing many of her official goddess duties, Hestia was a true homebody and the epitome of hospitality. Hestia was also responsible for keeping the hearth fires on Olympus burning perpetually, where she was rewarded with a seat and first choice of the offerings presented there.

Though by choice Hestia had no children of her own, new family members were presented to her at the hearth for her blessing and welcome into the home. She is portrayed as a humble woman whose main concern was domestic peace, to which she dedicated her time and talents.

Call on Hestia for no-drama solutions to family crises and evoke her energies to avoid them in the first place. She can also keep the fires burning within to motivate and spur you to action toward your goals. If standing true to your beliefs in the face of temptation or criticism is important, ask Hestia to walk quietly with you.

POWERS

Hestia was blessed with the gifts of inner fortitude, fire, and protection, keeping in mind fire is nourishing, but also destructive. Hestia gains strength from solitude and does not depend on others to fill her needs. She is steadfastly sure of herself, even when her norms go against the expected.

OFFERINGS

Not one for attention, simple offerings of food and a toast with wine at dinner in thanks Hestia will be pleased by. Offerings of California poppy, chaste tree, goldenrod, hollyhock, purple coneflower, and yarrow can help bring Hestia to your aid wherever domestic concerns lie.

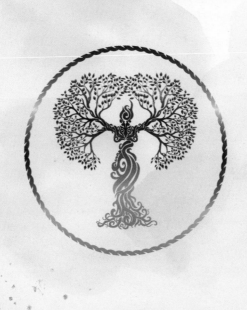

NIDRA (HINDU)

The beautiful Nidra Devi is goddess of the night and sleep, extolling the virtues of sound and restful sleep for the health of every human. She visits each night with her basket of dreams, which she gently empties over you just as divine sleep overtakes your mind and body. Those who live their lives true to their heart find sleep easily; those who don't, wait. Nidra lends her name to Yoga Nidra, a yogic practice leading to a sleep state of extreme relaxation between sleep and consciousness. It is said to be a powerful stress reliever.

Call on Nidra when the night's tossing and turning leave you tired, achy, foggy, and dreading another night of wakefulness, or when stress threatens to pull you under, but not to sleep.

POWERS

In addition to being able to sit with us in meditation to relieve stress and encourage sleep, Nidra also has the ability to help us manifest our truest wishes and bless us with good fortune. Her powers to grant peaceful sleep help sustain the energies of the world.

OFFERINGS

Water, for its soothing and purifying abilities, is the most valued gift to this goddess, as well as a clean altar on which to place it. Soothing music and a silent prayer honoring the sacred gift of sleep and gratitude for rest and renewal will help you form a solid bond with this goddess.

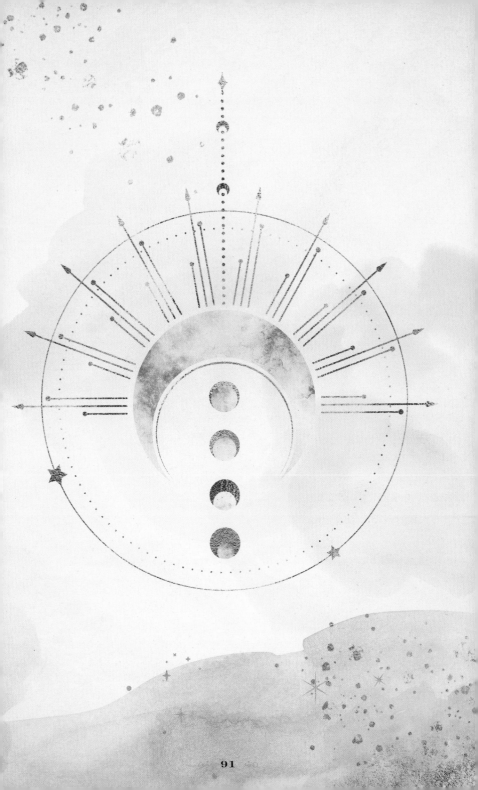

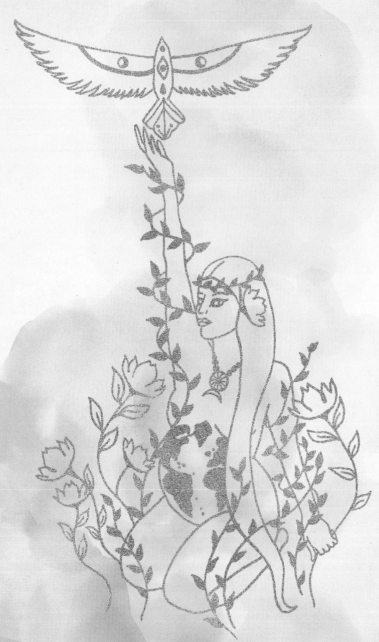

Pachamama, Andean goddess of abundance

Goddesses of Abundance, Good Fortune, and Prosperity

We all need a little help in the fortune, money, and luck arenas every now and then. These goddesses can help get you on your way to a more abundant, prosperous outlook. They can help nourish soul, body, and wallet.

The goddesses here are endowed with great wealth and a wealth of other virtues. They are generous of time, material goods, and spirits. Blessings of prosperity and luck flow easily from their energies. They will repay your acts of generosity multiple times over as well.

The gifts of these goddesses can increase many things in our lives besides money. They can also offer love, protection, hope, pleasure, freedom, and fertile energies—among others. Do not be selfish when dealing with these goddesses. While giving and kind, they expect honor and gratitude in return.

CELEBRATE THE GODDESS

Rejoice in your newfound friendships and celebrate the goddess. Honor her special days, work with her symbols, or just better appreciate her point of view with these tips and facts.

Berchta (Germanic), page 96

Berchta is celebrated from winter solstice, generally December 21, through the New Year—with a "Mother's Dinner." All work ceases in the home and fish soup is served in her honor. Ditch the housework and order takeout as a gift to Berchta.

Fortuna (Roman) / Tyche (Greek), page 97

June 24 marks the festival of Fors Fortuna, doubling this goddess's lucky charms. Offer a traditional toast of wine and count your blessings.

Lakshmi (Hindu), page 98

Goddess Lakshmi is honored during the yearly Diwali festival, the festival of lights. Draw a warm bath, surround yourself with candlelight, and prepare to celebrate with a relaxing goddess soak. Then, dress in your finest for a night out.

Pachamama (Andean), page 100

August 1 honors the abundance of Pachamama. Cook up a bounty and invite Pachamama to join you in celebration.

Rosmerta (Celtic), page 101

Mirroring Rosmerta's generous symbol of an overflowing cornucopia, place a bowl of fresh fruit on your table and give thanks for such easy access to nourishing food and clean water.

With goddess help, my heart expands—
ideas, intentions flow.

Join hand in hand, let's craft
a plan infused with fortune's glow.

Abundant blessings feed my dreams,
in fertile Earth they'll grow,

and echo life's most joyous song:
as above, then so below.

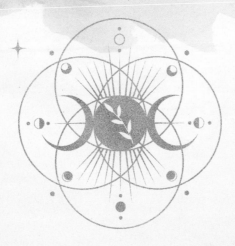

BERCHTA (GERMANIC)

A much-loved goddess of ancient Germanic origins, Berchta, who is also called Perchta, which means "bright," was the goddess of abundance and protector of the forest, animals, and of babies and children, especially of any unbaptized souls in the afterlife, which she nurtured in her beautiful garden. As goddess of abundance, it is said that offerings please Berchta so much, she returns the favor multiplied many times.

Her name is derived from the birch tree, with which she has a deep connection, along with evergreens, holly, flax, mayflowers, and wild berries. She is said to live among the forest, kept company by the snow, and is often pictured as a beautiful woman wearing a long, flowing white dress and white veil covering her face. Considered a Triple Goddess, she can take the form of maiden, mother, or crone. She often manifests with a webbed, goose-like foot, leading to the theory that she may have been the original Mother Goose. She is celebrated during Yule, a time when she arrives to chase away the cold of winter and to reward women for their hard work and good children with gifts—and punish those children who've been naughty.

Call on Berchta when restless ghosts of the past need to be tamed and transported to their final resting place so you can get on with the living, or when your generous spirit may be waning.

POWERS

Berchta's powers took the form of an abundant love and protection of children and in the ability to bring light to dark times. She recognizes and rewards good work and returns your generosity threefold.

OFFERINGS

Things familiar to Berchta will please her, like birch branches, anything white, beer, and traditional Yule treats, which originally had been left on rooftops in offering to her as she flew over on the winds in the Wild Hunt gathering lost souls.

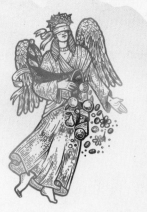

FORTUNA (ROMAN) / TYCHE (GREEK)

Fortuna may hail from as far back as the Etruscan civilization but was welcomed heartily by the Romans into their pantheon. If good luck is in your pocket, Fortuna—Lady Luck—is by your side. Historically, Fortuna was sought as a fortune-teller, with her response being delivered on a piece of paper nestled in a cookie (fortune cookie, anyone?)! Rumored to be the daughter of Jupiter, she inherited his bountiful traits. A cornucopia and wheel of fate are her symbols. Her Roman temple was fitted out with a horseshoe-shaped altar.

When working with Fortuna, take advantage of her generous nature and ability to bestow prosperity and abundance. Adored by mothers, Fortuna is particularly helpful in boosting fertile energies. She can help foretell the future, if that is what you wish—but beware the whims of fate, for happy outcomes are not always guaranteed and Fortuna likes to be in control of destiny.

POWERS

Luck, opportunity, wealth, and prosperity are the name of the game for Fortuna, as well as powers of divination. Concerning all her powers of abundance, Fortuna is generous to those she favors.

OFFERINGS

Fortuna smiles when any offerings are sent her way, but she particularly loves horseshoes, milk, and honey; sweet treats in round shapes, like her wheel of fortune; and a good game of poker in her honor.

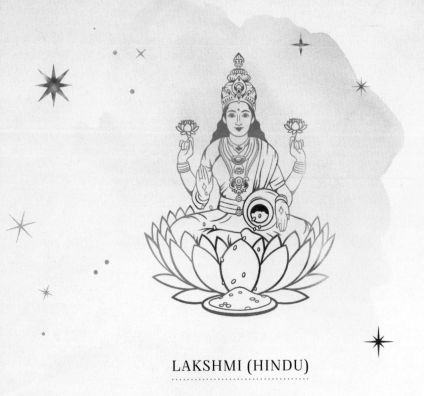

LAKSHMI (HINDU)

The Hindu goddess Lakshmi, partner to Vishnu, is goddess of
abundance, wealth, and prosperity. Believed to have emerged seated on
a lotus blossom from an ocean of milk churned in search of the nectar
of immortality, the beautiful Lakshmi is wealthy, kind, and generous.
She is often depicted with four arms, representing life's four inherent
values—*artha,* economy; *kama,* pleasure; *dharma,* honor; and *moksha,*
freedom—the achievement of which brings true fulfillment. She also
sits on a lotus blossom, whose message is one of transcending worldly
wealth for spiritual wealth, and the coins flowing from her hands
symbolize good luck and fortune, which are said to bless those whose
dwellings she visits.

Call on Lakshmi for help manifesting intentions born of a true
heart and sought with true desire. In more immediate matters, invoke
her name for some fortune and good luck on game day or any day your
luck feels a little dry.

POWERS

Lakshmi fosters spiritual as well as material wealth and increases fortunes through honorable means. Invite her into your realm for a boost of luck as well as financial reward. Her beauty radiates from her physical being as well as her generous spirit and kind soul. Seek her blessing when your world needs an extra bit of beauty and grace.

OFFERINGS

Beginning on a Friday, her day of worship, place a spell jar upon your altar next to a picture of Lakshmi, if you have one. Four times a day, for four days in a row, place four coins in your jar and give thanks to Lakshmi for her generosity and take a moment to be grateful for the abundance you enjoy and to visualize the wealth you desire. Create a beautiful altar to honor her and include red crystals, flowers, or candles (for the red silk robes she wears). Put lotus seeds, or lotus tea, in a dish and place next to a statue or picture of Lakshmi. Adding any special gifts that have great meaning to you is also appreciated.

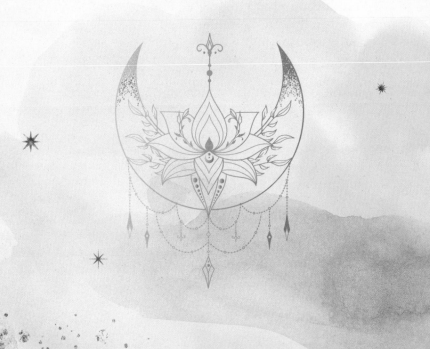

PACHAMAMA (ANDEAN)

Pachamama, Earth Mother and goddess of abundance, who took the form of a dragon and lived in the mountains, is worshipped by the People of the Andes as well as the Incas. She embodies the whole of the divine feminine and is at watch over issues of fertility, crops, and abundance. She represents the universe in its entirety, including time. Her powers of fertility here are vital to a bountiful harvest to sustain the people, and she provides everything necessary to sustain life. As protector, she guards against spiritual as well as material harm, but must be respected and honored to maintain the protective relationship. Worshippers believe earthquakes are Pachamama's response when she is slighted or feels no gratitude based on humans' disrespect of the land.

As Pachamama is the provider of all we need to live, call on her for any intentions you wish, but, as with manifesting all intentions, they must be true to your heart and your life. Invoke her especially when nourishment is required, whether it be spiritual, psychological, familial, or bodily.

POWERS

Pachamama's greatest power is to create, preserve, and sustain life. Her powers of love are transformative, yet celebrating her gifts is about unity with Earth. She is giver of life and helps us honor those who give life. Her wisdom allows us to see our place in the cosmos and take better care of it for future generations.

OFFERINGS

A few drops of beer or wine sprinkled onto the Earth to nourish it is a traditional offering to Pachamama. Any elements of the Earth in honor of Pachamama can accompany your sacred wishes; typically food and beer are offered. Connect with Earth in ways you may have left behind to honor Pachamama—swim in a pond, walk barefoot in the grass, blow dandelion wishes upon the breeze, or roast marshmallows over an open fire; all these represent some ideas to celebrate the element of water, Earth, air, and fire in her name. As a symbol of new life and growth, plant a tree.

ROSMERTA (CELTIC)

This powerful goddess of abundance, fertility, prosperity, and well-being was known as the Great Provider. Though Celtic in origin and widely revered, she was later also adopted and favored by the Romans. She carried a basket of fruit or overflowing cornucopia, offering plate and ladle, telling us of her generous nature and role as provider of prosperity. She is often depicted with a butter churn, thought to be symbolic of abundance, nourishment, and transformation, in the same way as the Celtic cauldron.

Call on Rosmerta to provide a fruitful harvest in whatever material activities you're invested—business, charity work, gardening, money, family fortune, and more.

POWERS

Rosmerta, the Great Provider, offers unending material sustenance, in whatever forms are needed, to those who worship her. She also possesses great healing powers and influence over Earth to produce bountiful harvests so all may be nourished and fed.

OFFERINGS

Spring water, as many of her shrines are associated with healing springs, and fresh fruit and vegetables are welcomed by Rosmerta.

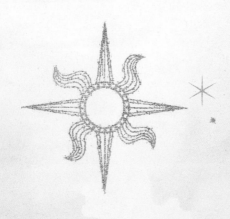

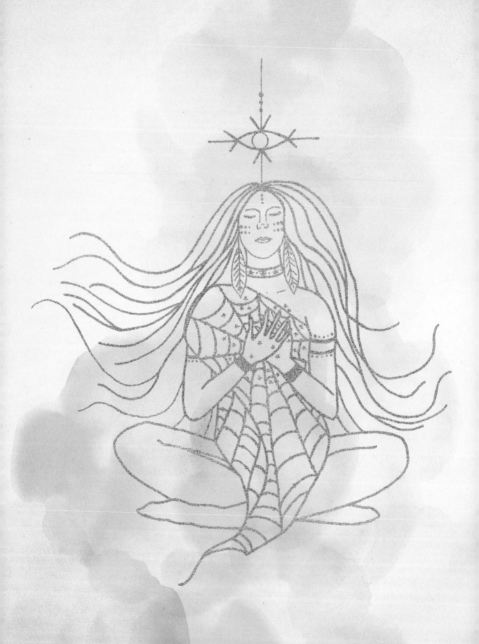

Spider Grandmother, Native American goddess of creation

Goddesses of Wisdom and Knowledge

The goddesses here possess the flames of eternal wisdom and knowledge—from the newness of creation to the wisdom of old age—and are eager to share their lessons with you.

These are goddesses whose powers reign supreme and whose knowledge is vast and varied—representing the original STEAM team (science, technology, engineering, arts, and math—or magic!). They can heal, nurture, guide, protect, teach, and help you survive. When life brings you to a crossroads, you'll have help deciding which path to take. They know herbs, and magic, and medicine. Their realms are of books, and buildings, and civilizations. Their energies are less emotional and more factual. They honor past, present, and future. You'll even find some lessons in manners along the way.

When working with these goddesses, bathe in their healing waters, listen to their wise counsel, and learn from their mistakes.

Give thanks for the time, trouble, and ill fortune they may save you from and give back by spreading your knowledge far and wide to help others manifest their dreams. Above all, recognize the talents of those who came before you, give thanks, and lift up others with your wisdom that their knowledge and wisdom may shine bright into the future.

CELEBRATE THE GODDESS

Rejoice in your newfound friendships and celebrate the goddess. Honor her special days, work with her symbols, or just appreciate her point of view more with these tips and facts.

ANAHITA (PERSIAN) / ANAITIS (GREEK), PAGE 106

With cultlike status, Anahita deserves adoration. Cleanse, bless, and decorate your altar accordingly.

SPIDER GRANDMOTHER (NATIVE AMERICAN), PAGE 107

A master weaver, Spider Grandmother would be honored if you learned or practiced the fiber arts, such as crochet, knitting, lacemaking, weaving, or embroidery.

HECATE (GREEK), PAGE 108

Every dark moon is a chance to visit Hecate, and the Esbat celebration of Samhain, October 31, the witch's new year, is prime. Connect with distant loved ones or honor those who have passed. Volunteer at an animal shelter, as Hecate loves dogs. Clean your closets and just let it go!

SESHAT (EGYPTIAN), PAGE 110

As Seshat is goddess of writing, write a letter on paper to someone you love. To honor her builder goddess status, build something: Legos with your kids, a model car or airplane, house of cards, sandcastles, whatever you fancy, and give thanks for the knowledge to do so.

SNOTRA (NORSE), PAGE 112

Mark the Esbat celebration of Mabon at the autumnal equinox, about September 21, honoring the harvest and hospitality. Have a party or just make someone feel special.

SOPHIA (GREEK) / HOKMAH (HEBREW) / SAPIENTIA (LATIN), PAGE 113

As Sophia is mother of Faith, Hope, and Charity, the best way to honor a mother is to compliment her children: Make a charitable gift with faith in others to do good works and for the hope it inspires.

With goddess sense of sight so keen
the darkness turns to light,

You're stirred to spread your wings aloft
with Full Moon shining bright.

Your wisdom comes with strength
to know when telling will delight,

Or guiding breeze needs whisper
sweet soft words of true and right.

O brilliant one who soars so deft
that not a sound is made,

Do help me see beyond the trees,
when guiding light does fade.

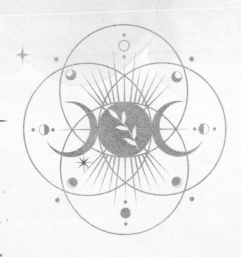

ANAHITA (PERSIAN) / ANAITIS (GREEK)

Anahita, also called Immaculate One, is a water goddess of wisdom and fertility and, like many powerful and richly revered goddesses, shares characteristics with goddesses of other cultures, such as Inanna and Venus. It is thought she may have originally been the same goddess as Saraswati and is hailed as a Great, or Mother, Goddess as well. Her exalted status may derive from the fact that she is identified as daughter of Ahura Mazda, Great Creator. Anahita is the source of all water on Earth—bringing with it healing, purification, and life itself, which allows wisdom to flow after. Her wisdom was especially useful in crafting victories from battle, and she was evoked by soldiers for just such favors. She is also, of course, beautiful and adorned with gold. Her chariot is pulled by four white horses: Cloud, Hail, Rain, and Wind.

Call on Anahita to clear and cleanse a chaotic mind, so wisdom may take its place. She can be particularly helpful in competitive situations where strategy begets victory, and in situations where preparing fertile ground for the birth of new ideas is needed.

POWERS

Anahita rules over healing waters, wisdom—closely associated with water—and fertility, and is guardian of women and their health. As a goddess of royalty, she blesses us all with the power of self-respect and permission to celebrate our divine inner goddess. With fertility her strongest asset, she breeds opportunities wherever she appears, tempered with the wisdom to use them wisely.

OFFERINGS

Clean water is the most meaningful offering to Anahita, including doing your part to keep Earth's water sources clean and plentiful. Roses, especially white, placed on your altar in her honor or in gratitude for her blessings are a lovely gesture.

SPIDER GRANDMOTHER (NATIVE AMERICAN)

Important to various Native American tribes, especially in the southwest United States, Spider Grandmother is a wise and nurturing figure who weaves the story of creation and time, and protects all she created—including the Sun and Moon. She spans the newness of creation and the wisdom of old age and, as such, is seen as both Earth goddess and crone goddess. She is respected as a teacher—to plant, to weave, to fashion pots from clay—and honored for her knowledge and survival skills. The interconnectedness of the threads of her world serves as a metaphor for magical living: one part cannot be touched without affecting another, as the ripples of energy travel through the web. Act only with positive intent.

Call on Spider Grandmother when fates may look decided but alternate paths are desired. Seek her counsel when faced with new beginnings and channel her patience to work to the end to manifest your dreams. Remember, it is bad luck to kill a spider—and its appearance may be a sign Spider Grandmother is weaving her protective web around you.

POWERS

Spider Grandmother demonstrates leadership, benevolence, creativity, courage, and survival. The power of her song brought life to her thoughts—and existence to the world. Her teachings are practical and her spirit indomitable.

OFFERINGS

Proper offerings for working with Spider Grandmother include cornmeal; bits of thread, wool, or woven materials; songs; clean earth on your altar; or a handmade piece of pottery. Stop to contemplate the intricate beauty of a spider's web in sunlight and give thanks for all creatures on Earth.

HECATE (GREEK)

Hecate was Triple Goddess of the Moon and the night, the spiritual world, magic, and crossroads—both symbolic and real. Guarding the ultimate crossroad, the border between life and death, Hecate can also carry messages back and forth between spirits and the living. She is capable of both good and evil and granter of both life and death.

Hecate is usually depicted with three heads, capable of looking in all directions at once: past, present, and future. Other manifestations of the Triple Goddess for Hecate are of Diana and Selene as maiden, mother, crone, and of the Moon—waxing, full, and waning. August 13 is the Day of Hecate.

As crone and dog-loving goddess of the waning and dark Moons, Hecate is often depicted carrying a torch—symbolic of her great wisdom. She used her immense knowledge and magical powers to benefit those who sought her help, and she is especially popular among witches for her magical skills and herbal healing knowledge.

Among her numerous associations are entrances; placing a shrine, or offering, to her at an entrance—whether to a structure or city—was believed to hinder evil spirits from entering.

Nighttime and the period during the Waning Moon are the best times to call on Hecate. Seek her aid in your magic work. Her wisdom is especially illuminating when it's time to step off your current path and forge a new path toward your goals. She can help you honor the past while living in the present and planning for the future. She can rid your world of ghosts, help secure victory in battle, and protect hearth and home. Encountering a dog, or hearing one bark, tells you Hecate has heard your plea.

POWERS

Hecate is immensely powerful. Her wisdom is deep, and her knowledge is wide. She is especially skilled in magic and revered for her knowledge and skills in herbal magic. To evoke Hecate is to instantly raise the energies and vibrations of your space.

OFFERINGS

Make your gifts and offerings at night. Cheese, bread, and eggs as well as food for her dogs are traditional for the "supper of Hecate," and are left at entrances or crossroads in her honor when seeking her favor. Garlic, lavender, honey, and willow (her traditional besom broom was bound with willow) are also dear to Hecate.

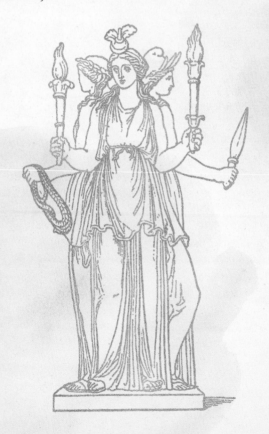

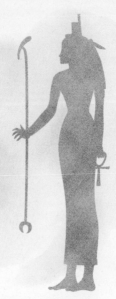

SESHAT (EGYPTIAN)

Goddess of wisdom, libraries, writing, and measurements, Seshat, lady of writing, was ruler of books and divine recordkeeper, tracking all aspects of ancient Egyptians' lives. Her father was Thoth (sometimes also her husband and counterpart, or brother, or both!), god of wisdom and time, and her mother was Ma'at, goddess of truth, justice, and universal order. Seshat is believed to have put her extraordinary skills with measurements to good use, helping the pharaohs build their magnificent temples—all perfectly aligned with the heavens to receive blessings from the gods—with the stretching of the cord ceremony, used to accurately measure and lay the foundation. As a result, she is also associated with mathematics and astrology. She was also gatekeeper of the afterlife, handing you your necessary travel documents to make safe passage. She was the embodiment of efficiency, list making, and accuracy. She is frequently seen carrying a palm stem, on which she marked off time.

Though particularly relevant to architects, Seshat can be of great help with all things requiring precise measurements for accurate results. Call on Seshat to bless your home library or help with an accounting class. Her list-keeping finesse can help boost your organizational skills and efficiency. Her observation skills at recording facts can help keep your own observations about events neutral and unbiased.

POWERS

As goddess of wisdom and knowledge, Seshat has useful and practical skills. She also has the power to grant pharaohs immortality, ascribing their names in the Tree of Life, and she honored the memory of those who passed by recording their life stories.

OFFERINGS

Special offerings to Seshat include journals, paper, pens, pencils— any books or writing instruments, really. She will particularly enjoy something you've written for her, especially a record of your ancestry.

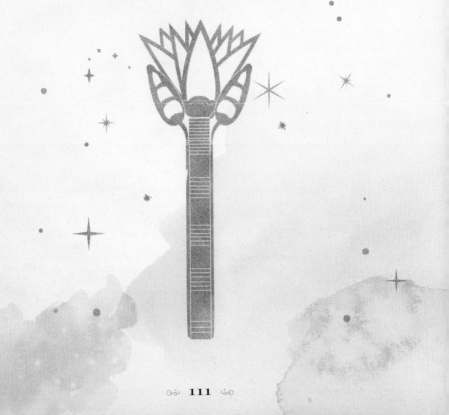

SNOTRA (NORSE)

Snotra is goddess of learning, wisdom, and hospitality, and especially of customs, courtesies, and manners. Snotra helps new goddesses adjust to their roles and seeks learning everywhere she looks. She collects the stories of her ancestors to learn from them and continue their legacy. She sees the good in all, no matter their bearing, and understands we all carry hidden burdens that a word of kindness can help ease. Disrespect of others or others' property does not sit well with her. She is known for building cairns atop a mountain with stones that she carries from bottom to top.

Snotra can be especially helpful at all kinds of gatherings where people may not know each other, such as weddings, business meetings, parties of all sorts, and meeting new colleagues. She's the stereotypical icebreaker who wants everyone to get along with ease and grace. She'll make sure everyone's glass is filled with praise and keep the conversation flowing.

POWERS

Snotra has the ability to make anyone feel comfortable and to help guide them through unfamiliar territory at ease. Her wisdom instructs the living and honors the lessons of her ancestors. She is a lifter of burdens and spirits.

OFFERINGS

Snotra appreciates all your efforts to make guests in your home feel welcome. She, with her exquisite manners, will gratefully accept any gifts or offerings made to her. Honor your ancestors. Learn a few words in another's language to make them feel seen. Place small piles of stones or crystals on her altar—and create an altar for her on a bookshelf filled with books.

SOPHIA (GREEK) / HOKMAH (HEBREW) / SAPIENTIA (LATIN)

Sophia is Gnostic goddess of wisdom—the source of wisdom and knowledge—and shines the light of knowledge on all who seek her. She is loving, giving, truthful, and protective, but also righteous. She also represents the divine feminine as she was adored as mother of the Universe. She is alternately paired with a god as co-creator or exiled from him, hidden to those others who wish to communicate with her, unless they search with a true heart.

When you take a moment to quiet the noise in your head and really listen to her wise and loving words, you'll thrive; ignore her at your peril. Truth is never to be feared from Sophia—it strengthens us—and she gives us the wisdom to listen compassionately, to find the truth in ambiguity. Faith, Hope, and Charity were her daughters, and with their mother, their story is one of speaking truth at any costs if it's what you believe and what you believe is right. Her symbol is a dove.

Call on Sophia when knowledge and truth can unite to strengthen your world and manifest your intentions. Seek her when fear of the unknown keeps you from acting. She can light the path forward with knowledge, dispelling fear and untruths along the way. Evoke her steadfastness to accomplish your goals.

POWERS

Sophia has the wisdom of the ages at her fingertips, tempered with compassion and faith. She embodies feminine power and is able to create much from little. Her rule over the righteous and just, combined with her wisdom, means prosperity for all who follow her ways.

OFFERINGS

Your presence is a gift to Sophia. Stay alert, as you may never know where you'll find her. Any objects of learning, such as books, or creation (think: the arts, gardening, food, writing) are welcomed by Sophia, as are generous acts to others in the name of her daughters. Images of doves on your altar can help you call Sophia to you.

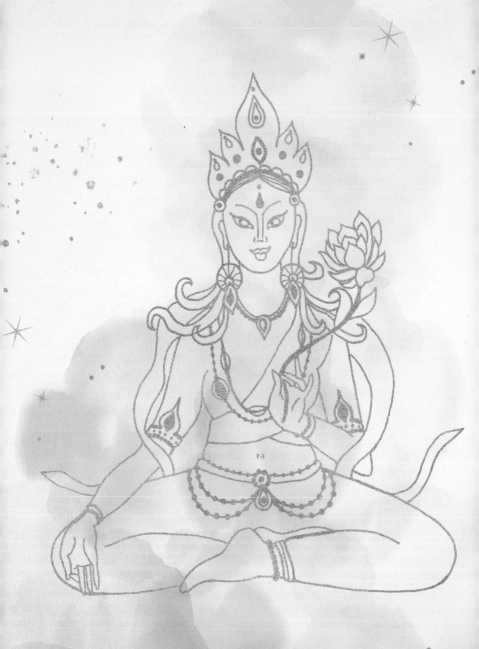

Tara, Hindu goddess of motherly love and protection

Goddesses of Strength and Protection

The Goddess Realm is full of fearless, courageous, powerfully protective allies. Some rely on pure strength and speed to accomplish their tasks, others on diplomacy or a fierce reputation. While here are just a few of the many empowering goddesses you may wish to know, they represent all that is good and strong about feminine love and wisdom when used to guard and protect loved ones.

Like all goddesses, you included, these can be contradictory in nature. They are typically independent and free-spirited in their approach to life—and fiercely protective, as you would expect, of all they love and rule over, and that passion spills over into other areas of their life. They are warriors, diplomats, activists for social and cultural change, and peacekeepers. You'll find many common characteristics with the undying strength and intuitive protection exhibited by Mother Goddesses, including the energies of love and compassion.

They can banish negativity, keep the peace—and keep evil spirits from your door. They will see you through hard work and cheer you with celebration on your achievements. They will protect you as you travel through life, and beyond. Work with these goddesses to help protect whatever is dear to you and draw on their strength to pursue your dreams.

CELEBRATE THE GODDESS

Rejoice in your newfound friendships and celebrate the goddess. Honor her special days, work with her symbols, or just better appreciate her point of view with these tips and facts.

Artemis (Greek) / Diana (Roman), page 119

August 13 is the Feast of Nemoralia, which honors Diana. Rituals included washing hair, then decorating it with flowers. Take a dip (or a bath) under a Full Moon and try out a new hairstyle to connect with this goddess.

Bastet/Bast (Egyptian), page 120

Earliest depictions of Bastet show her as a lioness; only later did she morph into the tamer version of a housecat. Any cat lovers should rejoice at the opportunity to bask in the Sun with Bastet to keep their claws sharp.

Durga (Hindu), page 122

Durga Puja, a multiday festival of Hinduism, celebrates good conquering evil and includes ceremonies, prayers, songs, and the building of pandals—highly decorated pavilions used to worship Durga. With its festival atmosphere as inspiration, organize a block party to honor Durga and all your goddess friends.

Lady Xian (Chinese), page 124

As diplomacy is Lady Xian's greatest weapon, worshippers come to her wishing for long happy lives, peace, and hopes for friendship around the world. Smile at a stranger; make a new friend; give someone a compliment in her honor.

Nike (Greek) / Victoria (Roman), page 125

April 12 celebrates this great goddess. Honor her gifts of strength and speed: Go for a run, a walk, a bike ride, a swim . . . just do it!

Tara (Hindu) / Sgrol-ma (Tibetan Buddhist), page 127

Tara is the personification of motherly love and protection. Honor all 21 aspects of Tara by giving bear hugs all around—and call your mother!

Goddess Realm of passion, strength,
and fearless courage, I pray:

Do clear the skies of threatening clouds
and corral the winds of change—

foretold by shifting energies,
whose strength repels the rains.

Protect me from the storms of life,
each one a lesson gained.

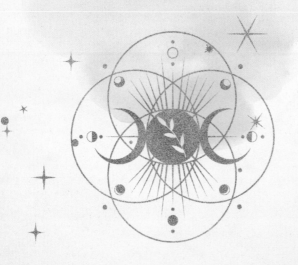

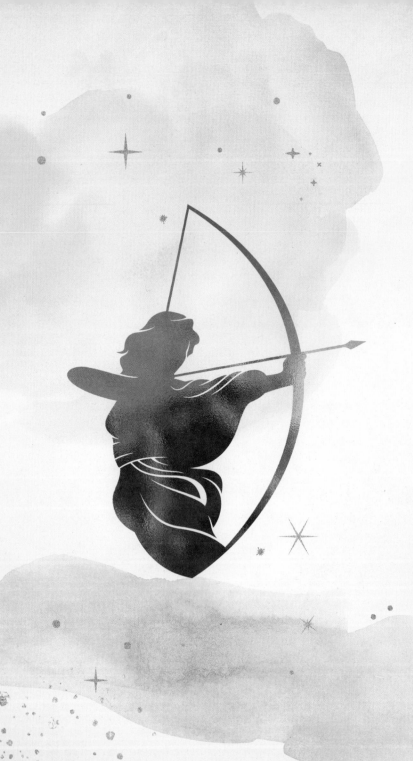

ARTEMIS (GREEK) / DIANA (ROMAN)

Artemis, goddess of the hunt, is a contradictory figure. In addition to the hunt, her realm included those wild animals she hunted, of which she was protectress; the forest; childbirth (born of assisting her mother's delivery of her twin brother, Apollo); virginity; and the Moon. Her role as guardian—of animals (the bear was sacred to Artemis), children, of her virginity, and easing suffering for older women—puts her in this category. Artemis was a free spirit, reveling in the mountains and forests while pursuing her delights. She lived on her own terms but was quick to show compassion to those needing it.

Call on the wisdom of Artemis when you want to feel empowered to achieve all you desire.

POWERS

Artemis was a supreme hunter, never missing her target. Her healing and protective powers, especially for children and against disease, were revered. She knew who she was and lived life accordingly, but with compassion and respect for others . . . unless they threatened what was important to her.

OFFERINGS

Moonstone offered during the Full Moon is an empowering offering. Add a statue of Artemis to your altar; adopt a pet; if you can, volunteer to clean a roadside. Place walnuts, figs, willow, artemisia, or tarragon on your altar as gifts.

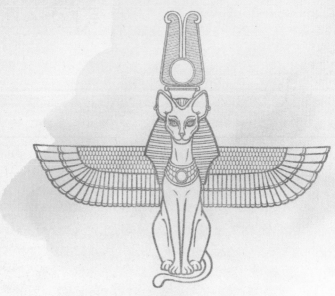

BASTET/BAST (EGYPTIAN)

This ancient Egyptian goddess of the rising Sun was extremely popular and widely celebrated—her annual festival was said to be quite spirited, similar to today's Mardi Gras. Bastet was a passionate protector of cats, women's secrets, home, and family, and goddess of all things pleasure, including music and dance—to name but a few of her Goddess Realms. Cats were significant in Egyptian culture as protectors of the crops—keeping the fields rodent-free, while helping to quell disease in this same way—and thought to be the physical manifestation of Bastet. She is also thought to have been goddess of the Moon. Not to be misunderstood, and very much catlike, she can be both gentle and fierce. Perhaps it's no surprise, but catnip was a sacred herb to Bastet—an offering cannot be resisted. Bastet also had associations with fertility and childbirth as well as perfumes and ointments.

Call on Bastet when a little feline influence might add a sense of play to your life, or when the claws need to come out in the form of defense and protection. Working with Bastet can keep health, home, and hearth all in good order—and evil spirits from your doorstep.

POWERS

Bastet's powers of protection reign supreme, especially of women and children, and keeping disease and evil spirits from the home. She also has the power of knowing how to kick up her (kitten) heels and have a good time.

OFFERINGS

Bastet adores anything cat related, and especially catnip—so, why not adopt a cat, if you can! Wine, music, and dance celebrate her goddess stature. In addition, moonstone will help call forth her Moon goddess qualities for you, and yellow candles, in honor of her association with the Sun, honor Bastet. Wearing your favorite perfume in her presence will establish a connection.

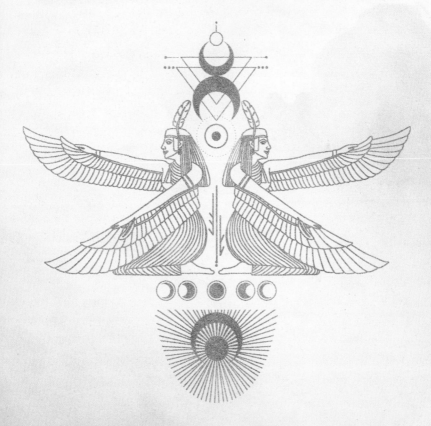

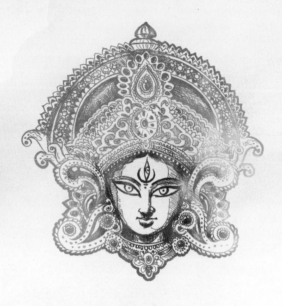

DURGA (HINDU)

Though known as a warrior goddess, Durga, which means "invincible," is also known as Shakti or Devi, and is the universal mother protector and keeper of the peace. She symbolizes the divine feminine energy in use against forces of evil. As are all mothers, Durga is a supreme multilimbed multitasker—ready to respond to threats of any kind in any direction at any time. As well as her many limbs, her three eyes give her great power. The left eye, the Moon, represents desire or intent; her right eye, the Sun, is action; and the middle eye, fire, is great knowledge. Among the many weapons she carries in her eight arms to enact battle are a trident (courage), lotus (a sign of victory, but not without hard work), and thunderbolt (steadfastness of convictions). Durga navigates the world riding a fearsome lion, demonstrating her courage, control, power, and leadership.

Call on Durga to battle external evil as well as the negative forces and fears that lurk inside you. If you put your faith in her, she will be there to protect, defend, and teach you her strategy for winning the battles that bring on real change.

POWERS

Durga's power lies in battling evil and negative forces that threaten the peace, prosperity, and well-being of those she protects. She has the power to grant peace, cleanse your spirit, and renew positive energy when petitioned for such.

OFFERINGS

Anything red, which is the traditional color of her sari, will please and appease this goddess. The hibiscus flower is a traditional gift.

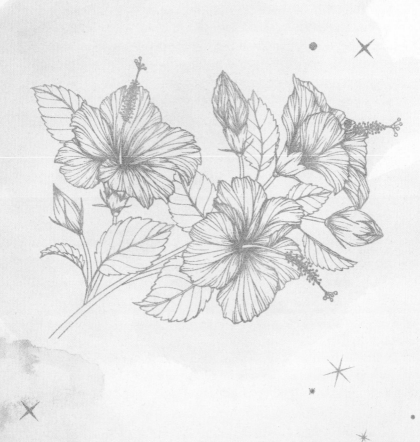

LADY XIAN (CHINESE)

Lady Xian was a Chinese nobleperson born in 512 CE. She developed into a fierce protector of her people and promoter of peace among tribes, relying on negotiation and diplomacy versus weapons and war. She was a revered local leader, in a time when women were not, and was fair and just—but strict and impartial in handing down punishments when deserved. Lady Xian was a warrior, diplomat, activist for social and cultural change, and peacekeeper. She lived a long life, serving emperors through the Liang, Chen, and Sui dynasties, earning her much praise and the adoration of a deity for her loyalty, courage, and dedication to protecting her people.

Call on Lady Xian to protect in times of uncertainty in ways that lead to unified agreement and positive change. Ask her for courage and guidance when conflict looks inevitable, or action is needed to protect and preserve what's most valuable to you. Ask her to lend you her voice when speaking truth to power is required.

POWERS

Lady Xian wielded confidence, courage, and diplomacy as her weapons against evil. Never underestimate the power of one person to positively affect the lives of many, or be afraid to use your powers for the good of others.

OFFERINGS

Lady Xian valued loyalty above all—be prepared to develop a relationship with her and she will reward you handsomely. Offerings of items of personal value, such as trophies or other awards you have earned, will please her, as will any symbol from your culture that speaks of peace, such as an olive branch.

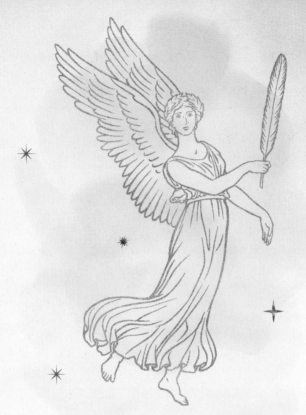

NIKE (GREEK) / VICTORIA (ROMAN)

Nike, or winged goddess, is the Greek goddess of strength and victory and was one of the first volunteers to join Zeus's army to fight against the Titans, where she was appointed chief chariot driver. Their victory in battle earned her a permanent residence on Olympus with him afterward. The goddess is often depicted winged, marking her speed, agility, and ability to adapt to changing circumstances at a moment's notice. She is frequently seen carrying a palm branch in one hand, a sign of victory and the peace it brought, and a laurel wreath in the other for crowning the next victor—eager to give credit where credit is due. Nike loved a toast, a song, and a dance as the victory lap for any achievement earned.

Call on Nike when the battles just seem too tough to go alone, or your goddess energy is not enough to sustain you through the battle.

POWERS

Nike was worshipped for her gifts of strength and, especially, speed, making her victorious in any battle, competition, or daily struggle, which she could also bestow on others as she pleased—but be forewarned: If you were deemed not worthy, the victory was snatched away. Her speed granted her the power to hover over battlefields, taking in all perspectives and quickly adjusting tactics.

OFFERINGS

Nary a general, soldier, or serious athlete went into battle without first offering a prayer to Nike. Once victory is achieved, wine, laurel or palm branches, and proof of achievement are fine thanks for Nike's help.

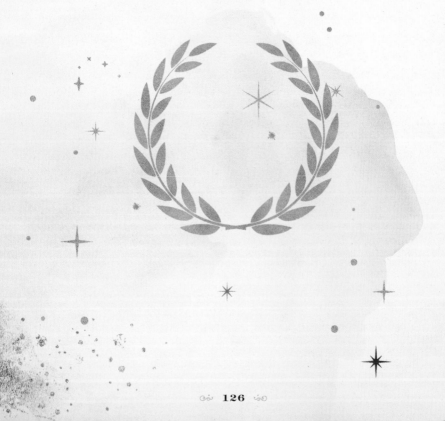

TARA (HINDU) / SGROL-MA (TIBETAN BUDDHIST)

Tara is one of the oldest goddesses still worshipped today and is the most popularly worshipped goddess in the Tibetan pantheon. Originating as a life-giving Mother Goddess, Tara, whose name means "star," is a protective goddess of travel, both earthly and spiritual, as we move through life. She is the feminine counterpart to the bodhisattva (enlightened one) Avalokiteshvara, and is said to be born of a lotus flower, rising in a lake formed from his tears of compassion while witnessing the world's suffering. There are 21 manifestations of Tara, with the White Tara and the Green Tara being most well known. The White Tara is a gentle, compassionate protectress who comes in peace, whereas the Green Tara is a fiercely protective goddess willing to do what it takes to save us from harm.

Call on Tara when you feel the need to protect those you love and to channel her caring, compassionate ways when enduring stressful times.

POWERS

Tara's great powers lie in her deep well of compassion and willingness to fiercely protect those she loves. Her tireless work on behalf of all humanity and her wisdom to guide our transformative journeys are why she is worshipped.

OFFERINGS

Seek Tara's favor and guidance with offerings of lotus blossoms, anything star-star shaped, or green or white crystals such as jade, emerald, peridot, diamond, clear quartz, or selenite. White and green candles on your altar make appropriate tools to indicate your intentions to Tara.

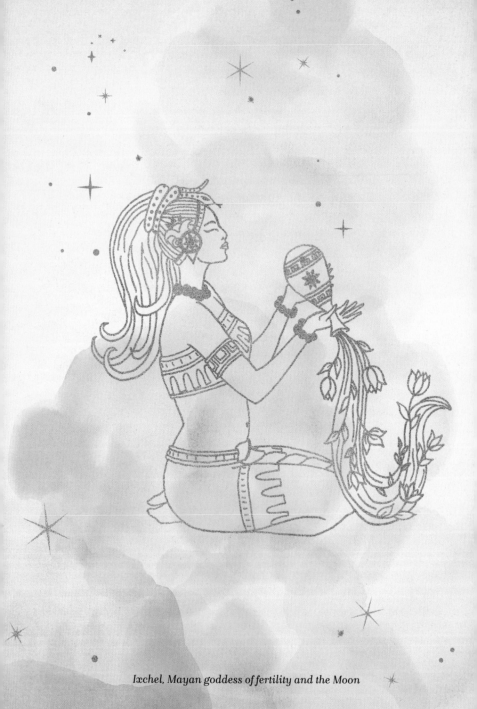

Ixchel, Mayan goddess of fertility and the Moon

Goddesses of Creativity and Joy

Living joyfully is something to strive for every day, and this group of goddesses leads the way in highly creative fashion. These goddesses are not simply creative for creativity's sake, but also know the value of their talents and how to use them for the good of achieving outcomes and helping humanity. Home crafts, music and arts, strategy, and persuasion are but some of the talents discovered here. Known for their ability to bring joy and celebration to life, they can inject life into any party. And there is always one in the crowd who can make you laugh out loud despite yourself. You'll find no self-consciousness in this group—just a pure lust for life and all that makes it a joy to live.

And, perhaps, in the unlikeliest of places, you'll perceive messages of self-acceptance, strength, and the ability to laugh at yourself.

Travel with these goddesses, exploring all that lies within. Learn about letting go and fresh starts and grace under pressure. Find the beauty in all that surrounds you. Name a festival in your honor. Let your creativity flow when in their company and see what happens.

CELEBRATE THE GODDESS

Rejoice in your newfound friendships and celebrate the goddess. Honor her special days, work with her symbols, or just better appreciate her point of view with these tips and facts.

Athena (Greek) / Minerva (Roman), page 133

Panathenaea was the ancient festival held in June to honor the multitalented Athena on her birthday, and where you could find everything from chariot races to gymnastics competitions, and musical and equestrian contests. Use whatever talents you have that Athena has blessed to honor her.

Hathor (Egyptian), page 134

The annual Hathor Festival, July 19, celebrates her birthday. Devotees were encouraged to party it up in her honor. Do so responsibly in your honor. Bread and beer please, Hathor.

Baubo/Iambe (Greek), page 138

What's better than a belly laugh and a good (dirty!) joke? Don't wait for a special occasion to seek Baubo's company . . . laugh every day, make someone smile, tell a good joke, watch a funny movie. It's good for you.

Ixchel (Mayan), page 136

Honor Ixchel, Lady of the Rainbow, by burning candles on your altar in a rainbow of colors, especially orange for its creative energies. Better yet, honor her Mayan ancestors, who believed the cacao bean had magical powers, by eating some chocolate, too.

Laetitia (Roman), page 139

Laetitia was famously depicted on numerous coins both in her honor and to spread happiness among the people. Some retail therapy is likely in order to channel Laetitia's joy.

The Muses (Greek), page 140

To connect to these Greek goddesses of the arts, music, dance, poetry, literature, science, and knowledge, organize a trip to your local museum to appreciate all the talent inspired the world over by these lovelies.

Saraswati, also Sarasvati (Hindu) / Benzaiten (Japanese), page 142

Vasant Panchami, or Saraswati Puja, is a popular Hindu spring festival dedicated to this goddess. Traditions include dressing up in yellow and giving yellow treats to friends and family in celebration. Make some lemon bars and share the joy.

The Three Graces (Greek), page 145

These three sisters spread goodwill and joy wherever they found themselves. In their honor, organize a girls-only weekend, call your sister, or pay it forward to make someone's day.

Your face never ceases to inspire me.

Your words never cease to guide me.

Your arms never cease to assure me.

Your charms never cease to enchant me.

Connected to you, dear goddess, I feel loved, I feel capable.

I feel joy. I feel free.

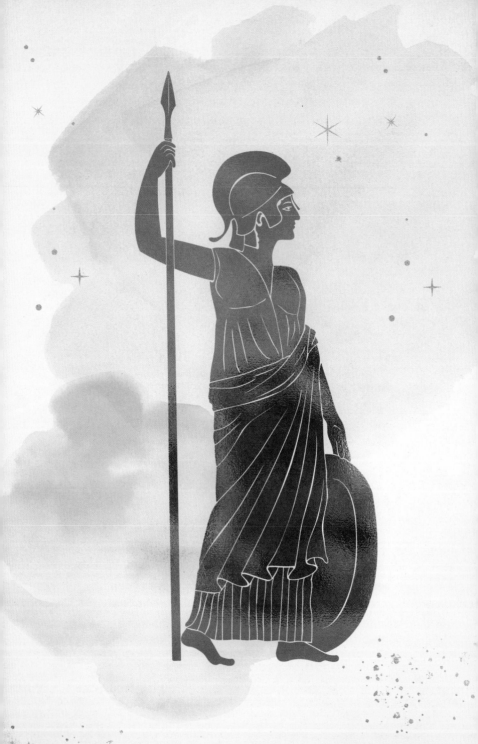

ATHENA (GREEK) / MINERVA (ROMAN)

Goddess of crafts, as well as wisdom, courage, protection, and war, Athena was one of the most creative of the Olympian goddesses—said to have been born fully grown and dressed for battle! In her role as goddess of handcrafts, she was patron of all the arts and a builder who bestowed the more practical gifts of cooking and sewing to mortals. The great temple Parthenon was built to honor Athena. Her gift to the Greeks, the olive tree—with its symbolism of peace—was sacred to her, as was the oil created from the fruit it bore. Bearing her seemingly contradictory roles with grace and inspiration, she formed the foundation of civilization's growth. Athena was the supreme balance of masculine and feminine, promoting the thriving, independent survival of women in a man's world and relishing in a woman's strength to serve. She is often depicted with an owl.

Call for Athena when strength and courage wane and the ability to manage conflicting priorities is a burden. Seek her inspiration and ideas when tackling new projects or when the gift of persuasion is needed to succeed. Use her warrior goddess persona to fuel the passion you have and to bolster the courage to take risks and harness the creativity needed to achieve your dreams.

POWERS

Athena uses her creativity to invent practical, useful solutions to problems. Her intelligence and strategic-thinking skills allowed her to navigate the trials of war and the ability to make peace with equal ease. She is also a shape-shifter, able to assimilate herself into situations to influence outcomes without being detected or recognized.

OFFERINGS

Olive oil, music, wine, and honey make effective offerings, as do handwoven and handmade objects—anything made from our own hands and talents.

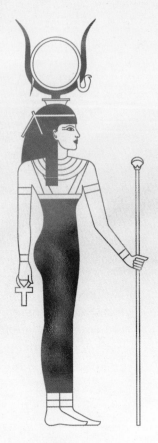

HATHOR (EGYPTIAN)
....

Many of the goddesses throughout time have been supreme
multitaskers, enjoying status and reign over numerous areas. The same
applies to Hathor, the ancient Egyptian cow-headed goddess, frequently
worshipped as a Mother Goddess and nourisher, ruler of the Sun, Moon,
and Sky, and revered for her powers of rebirth and light. She is included
in this category, however, because of her simultaneous association
with joy, song, dance, celebration, and gratitude. Originally sent by Ra
to wreak havoc and destruction on all of humanity in punishment for
its ungratefulness, Hathor transforms into the crazed and vindictive
Sekhmet, and thus, is associated with the Eye of Ra. Ra, however, having

recognized the faulty plan he put into motion, gets Sekhmet drunk on a special batch of beer. Sekhmet falls asleep and awakens as the beautiful, benevolent Hathor.

Seek Hathor to bring joy and celebration to your days and inspire gratitude for all in your life that makes you happy. She can also help you get your feminine side in groove when your self-esteem is feeling a bit sidelined.

POWERS

As a goddess, Hathor's power was in all things feminine and had influence over every area of life and death. She is depicted in an early personification of the Milky Way, as it was thought sweet milk flowed from the udders of the heavenly cow goddess. Her joyous association with song and dance can inject the life into any party.

OFFERINGS

In the tradition of the Five Gifts of Hathor, write down five things you are grateful for and place them on your altar, or safely burn the list as you give silent thanks for Hathor's benevolence. An aura of gratitude lifts the cloud of depression. Other welcome gifts include a mug of beer, a glass of milk, copper or turquoise items, and sycamore tree leaves. Wearing make-up is seen as a sign of worship for Hathor, and gifts of mirrors to reflect her beauty are encouraged.

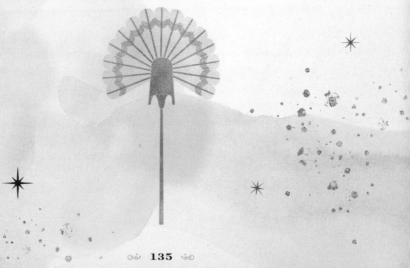

IXCHEL (MAYAN)

With a name meaning "lady rainbow," the beautiful Triple Goddess
Ixchel is goddess of fertility and childbirth—both highly creative
undertakings as well as signs of new beginnings—who reigns over
creativity in all its forms, which she demonstrated in her extraordinary
weavings. Like the soothing water she is associated with, Ixchel is
goddess of the Moon, waxing and waning from beautiful young maid
to crone throughout the Moon's phases, and can release the flow of
creativity in you.

Her story is one of chasing unrequited love, only to catch it and
find it not as loving as she thought. Taking matters into her own
hands (but not before being struck and killed by lightning sent by her
grandfather—then coming back to life after 13 days of attendance by
grieving dragonflies!), Ixchel recognized what she could not change,
and so she disappeared into the night sky, taking the form of a jaguar,
and chose a newly creative life using her talents to help others. Ixchel is
often pictured with a rabbit, a figure the Mayans, like the Chinese, saw
in the face of the Moon, and is a symbol of fertility.

Call on Ixchel when letting go of something to make room for a
new start, or do so at the start of any new project to encourage fresh
ideas that can get the creative juices flowing. Seek her wisdom when
challenges beset you and listen to her soothing words to deal with them
with grace and perseverance. Practice self-care in her honor.

POWERS

Ixchel is a supremely wise goddess. Through her continuous cycle of
rebirth, she sees the mysteries of all seasons of life and can help you
see them as well. As goddess of water and lady of the rainbow, Ixchel
sent rains to nurture crops and deliver the harvest. Her skills as a
weaver can help you weave together the life you desire. When you spy a
rainbow, acknowledge her presence.

OFFERINGS

Seek Ixchel's grace and blessing with offerings of clean water, moonstone, a prism, anything blue, or symbols related to the Moon, rabbits, jaguars, or dragonflies. Incorporate fresh herbs or pomegranate juice or seeds into your kitchen routine, or place a jar of healing herbs or a rainbow-colored bouquet of flowers on your altar as a symbol of gratitude and to call her to your side.

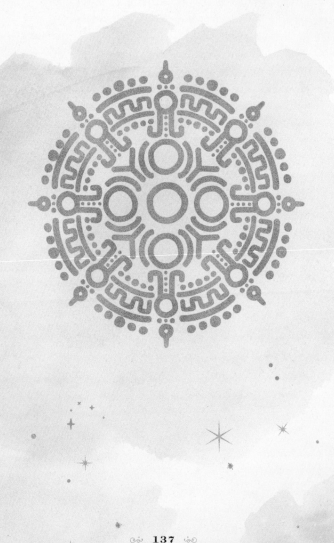

BAUBO/IAMBE (GREEK)

Baubo, also known as Iambe, was born to Pan and Echo. The meaning of her name is disputed, but one translation is "belly," or "belly laugh." She was considered the goddess of mirth and good humor—more than often a bit lascivious. Her reputation for such began when she first delighted and cheered the grieving Demeter, who was in frantic search of her daughter, Persephone, with bawdy jokes and a dance—purportedly lifting her dress to the amusement of all (perhaps the original cancan girl?). She was also known for her sometimes biting wit. Baubo stands guard as protector of women and children and, importantly, is viewed as a powerful example of promoting positive body image.

Evoke Baubo when lightening the mood can defuse emotions or when seeking the poetry her alternative name inspires to cleverly craft your message. Listen to Baubo's wisdom of self-acceptance when that negative self-talk just won't quit. Her words have power and can bring a smile to your face and healing to your heart. Most of all, never be afraid to laugh at yourself.

POWERS

Baubo's powers lie in her enormous laugh, her creativity, and the ability to see the humor in any situation, and as such, she also has the tremendous healing power that laughter brings. Her ability to read a situation and intuit the best course of action is something we all aspire to. She also possesses one of the greatest powers of all—self-love and acceptance.

OFFERINGS

Not surprisingly, Baubo loves a good joke and a hearty laugh. Music to dance by and songs to sing are also appropriate offerings, as well as anything funny, silly, or lighthearted.

LAETITIA (ROMAN)

Roman goddess of joy and celebration, Laetitia is associated with holidays and festivals. Her name means "happiness"—especially concerning prosperity and plenty. She is often depicted wearing a wreath or garland of leaves, flowers, or branches, the traditional sign of celebration and honor—such as we use for our Christmas holidays and to honor other celebrations and special occasions. She is pictured frequently with a ship's rudder, signifying her guiding actions in matters of good fortune.

Call on Laetitia in matters of money that can solve problems and create ease and joy in your life—but don't overlook the emotional benefits of happiness and celebration she can also bring to your world.

POWERS

Laetitia spreads joy and celebration wherever she goes and can turn any day into a festive occasion. Her joy is not frivolous, though, as each person's joy results from different needs being met. She teaches us to be joyous in all circumstances, even in times of need.

OFFERINGS

Because Laetitia was depicted so frequently on coins, any coin is a worthy offering. Food gifts, representing the symbol of food abundance as a sign of wealth, honor Laetitia. Wreaths and garlands made of flowers or greenery represent her festive nature. Anything yellow, the color of happiness, is also a good idea.

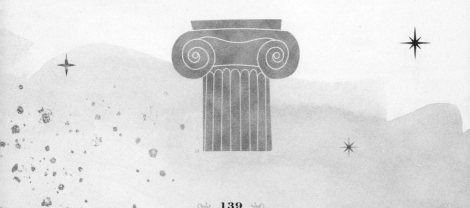

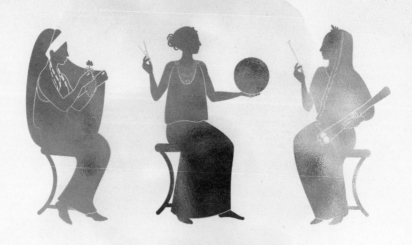

THE MUSES (GREEK)

The Muses, of which there are nine, are Greek goddesses of the arts: music, dance, poetry, literature, science, and knowledge. Their gifts of the arts were also gifts of joy—and like all goddesses, they possessed great beauty. The Muses inspired all artists to reach their greatest potential—but they were not to be challenged as to their supreme reign in the arts, or else trouble ensued. They entertained the Olympian gods and their works were of such perfection they were said to make you forget all troubles (perhaps as an antidote to their mother, Mnemosyne, goddess of memory, who would not let you forget anything!).

Align your talents and intentions with a favorite muse. Calliope—epic poetry; Clio—history; Erato—love poetry; Euterpe—music; Melpomene—tragedy; Polyhymnia—sacred hymns; Terpsichore—choral song and dance; Thalia—comedy; and Urania—astronomy.

POWERS

The Muses are immense sources of creative inspiration and a font of knowledge in times of need, serving not just poets, writers, and musicians but thinkers of all types. Their gifts may be granted at random, so be aware and be ready to take action if you ask for their help. They also have the ability to entertain and distract a stressed mind from its burdens.

OFFERINGS

Honey and milk will delight all The Muses, but you can also make offerings appropriate to the specific Muse you're working with, for example: a poem to any of The Muses associated with poetry; music to the musically inclined Muses; a good joke for Thalia; a section in your journal dedicated to your time with Clio. Whatever The Muses inspire in you, the gift of gratitude and the sharing of your talents are key.

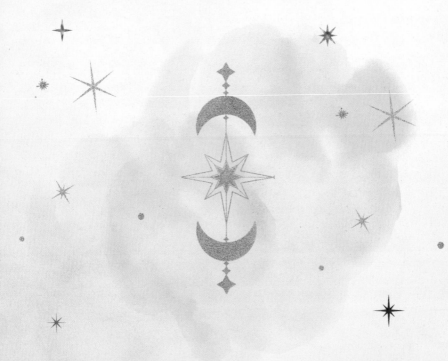

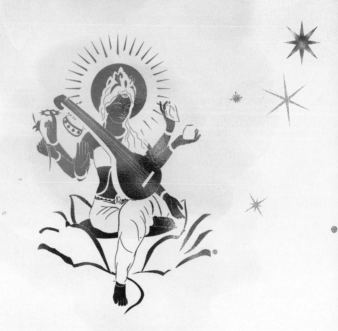

SARASWATI, ALSO SARASVATI (HINDU) / BENZAITEN (JAPANESE)

Mother of the Vedas, goddess of learning, music, art, and wisdom, and consort of Brahma, Saraswati is also credited with having invented Sanskrit and teaching the god Ganesh to write. Her name means "flowing" and she is the personification of the sacred river Sarasvati, source of cleansing and good fortune to all those who take to her waters. The free flow of the good fortunes of wisdom and consciousness all come from her, as do the flowing gifts of water, words, and knowledge. Saraswati is a member of a female trinity (including Lakshmi, see page 98, goddess of wealth, and Parvati, goddess of love) that works together to keep the Universe—created by their male counterparts—in order.

    Call on Saraswati when the pressure is on for a good performance—whether of the musical variety, educational testing, or that coveted job interview, or when her gift of eloquence can help convey your true thoughts.

POWERS

If you listen carefully when working with Sarasvati, you'll hear the tunes she plays on her traditional stringed *veena*, which accompany us through life. She can teach you the true wisdom in your heart and give you the tools to express your creativity to the world, especially as a musician or writer.

OFFERINGS

Give offerings to Saraswati with books, pens, musical instruments, and white-colored items, especially silk, which Saraswati is often shown wearing while riding her white swan or seated on a white lotus blossom.

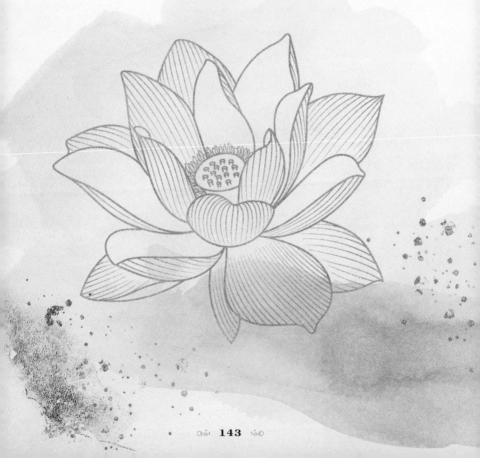

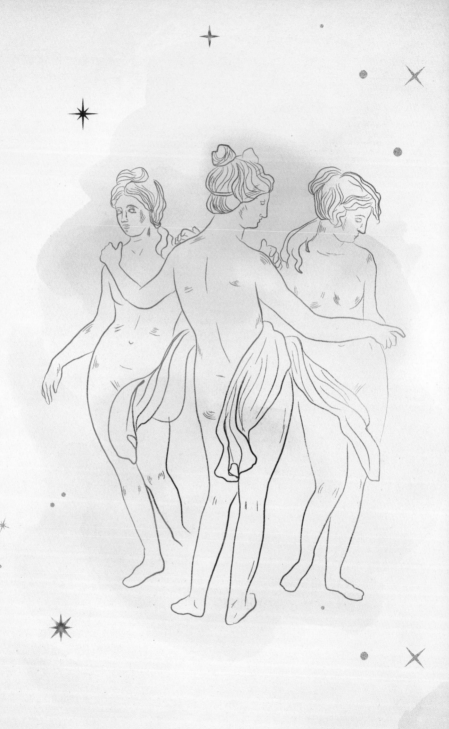

THE THREE GRACES (GREEK)

The Three Graces were goddesses of mirth, beauty, and charm, tasked with bringing joy to the world—and to protect such as well. They were the veritable "cruise directors" of ancient life, seeing to everyone's pleasure and entertainment. Aglaia (splendor), Euphrosyne (joy), and Thalia (blossoming) were the life of the party. The first cup of wine is always offered in toast to them.

Call on the Three Graces when your world needs a little boost of beauty or spark of joy to ignite a fresh, new, positive attitude.

POWERS

The powers of the Three Graces manifest in the ability to be "grace" under pressure, see the beauty in everything—no matter how small— and put the happiness and welfare of others ahead of your own.

OFFERINGS

Any fresh flowers—especially roses—wine, dance, song, and living a joyful life are special offerings you can make to the Graces. Finding the beauty in the everyday and unexpected is a gift to them as well as yourself, and will bring much happiness in return.

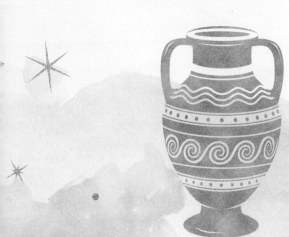

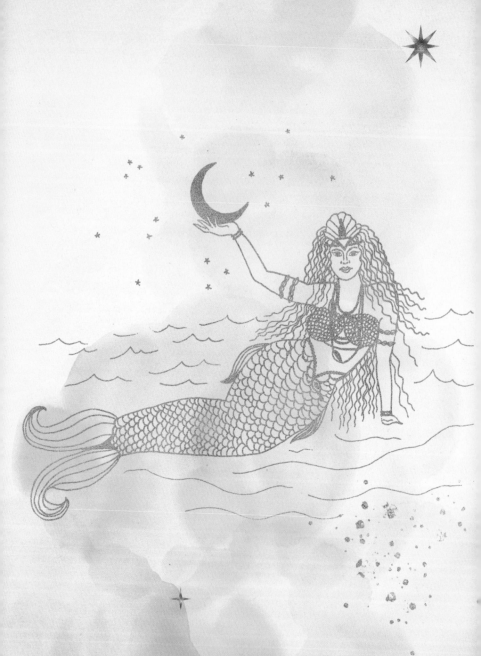

Yemaya, Yoruban Mother Goddess and water spirit

Goddess Magic Spells and Rituals

The Goddess Realm is here for you whenever you feel the need. Calling upon goddess energy for spellwork and rituals is like placing a magnifying glass over the particular power you're seeking—it boosts the energy intensely and draws it from within you. When aligned with your intentions and released into the Universe, goddess magic occurs. But remember, the intentions must be true, and the heart must believe. It is also a way to honor your true spirit.

Other than goddess energy, the natural energies of crystals, herbs and flowers, candles (fire), color, and essential oils—some of the items you might choose to dress your altar with (see page 13)—can also amplify energies to manifest results. In all, use what speaks to you and feels right.

The Moon, too, is of particular importance in spellcasting— particularly if working with a goddess associated with this wondrous object—as it is a revered source of heightened intuition. The Moon's waxing (growing) phases, from New Moon to Full Moon, are powerful for pulling things to you; the waning (diminishing) phases, from Waning Gibbous to Waning Crescent, then starting again with the New Moon, can be a strong ally in letting things go.

Taking care and time to connect to your goddess leaves you fiercely powerful to accomplish all that you desire!

SUMMONING GODDESS MAGIC
AND SPELLCASTING TIPS

Spells can be personal or universal, depending on the circumstances and need. Casting spells can be as formal or informal as you like and, as stated previously, does not require any tools or equipment except you, your intentions, and belief. Rituals are usually a bit more elaborate than spells and, again, do only what feels right for you. I've kept things simple here. Feel free to embellish as your experience, desire, and creativity inspire you.

When casting spells, here are a few basic guidelines to use or adjust to make them your own. A few calming and centering breaths to start are always welcome. Then:

- Know your intentions. Be what you want to manifest.

- Prepare your altar and any tools you're using.

- Cast a circle around your sacred space in which to work—whether by strewing dried herbs that support your intentions, placing crystals in a circle on your altar or around you with salt or eco-friendly glitter (great outside!), or simply drawing a circle in the air with your finger. Remember to release the circle when you've finished.

- Visualize the outcomes you desire.

- Make an offering and call for your goddess.

- Cast your spell.

- Believe in the energy of love and healing.

- Visualize your goddess saying goodbye.

- Be grateful and give thanks.

WEAVING THE GODDESSES INTO YOUR MAGICAL LIFE

There are so many ways to honor and respect the goddesses as part of your magical life. Whatever you choose, make it as ritualistic or as simple as you like—have fun with it and consider any activity you do as a way to unleash your goddess magic! Understanding a bit about each goddess and her personality, powers, associations, and preferences is the easiest way to start. The more you the learn about them, the more ideas you'll develop to work with them. Here are some suggestions to set you on your goddess path.

If a goddess is associated with:

- **AIR:** *Wear a feather; let the breeze carry away your wishes; open a window to refresh a room.*

- **ANIMALS:** *Get a pet; volunteer at a shelter; delight in Nature's creatures; donate to an animal charity.*

- **CREATIVITY:** *Laugh; learn a craft; redecorate a room or your altar; paint, sing, dance, write, recite poetry; learn a language; daydream.*

- **EARTH:** *Take a walk in Nature; sit barefoot in the grass; plant a garden; visit a farmers market; eat mindfully; host a harvest dinner for friends and family.*

- **FIRE:** *Light a fire in your cauldron or a candle on your altar; sit in front of a fireplace, campfire, or other source of heat; gaze at the sunset.*

- WATER: *Incorporate water activities into your life, like ritual bathing; swim in the ocean, a pond, stream, or pool; cook; practice ritual cleaning; make Moon water and use it for blessings, altar offerings, teas; make snow angels; go ice skating.*

- FERTILITY AND MOTHERHOOD: *Lift up others; show unconditional love for all—yourself included; celebrate all that is bountiful in your life.*

- HERBS: *Plant an herb garden; cook with fresh and dried herbs; hang an herb wreath in your kitchen; share recipes with friends and list the meanings and associations of the herbs used.*

- FLOWERS AND TREES: *Hold a tree-planting ceremony; plant a garden; bring fresh flowers into the house for their beauty and healing energies.*

- THE AFTERLIFE: *Honor your ancestors; let go of what no longer serves.*

Spells and Rituals

To make calling for the goddesses' attention and energy a bit easier, here you'll find spells and rituals covering many of the aspects for which you may seek help. Never hesitate to use your own words, as truth spoken from the heart is the most beautiful magic of its own.

In the end, take what you need, give what you can, be kind, be grateful. The positive energy you send out with your spells will be returned to you multiplied—just not always when expected or desired. Be patient and believe.

And remember: Magic is all around you and there whenever you need it—but the Universe gives us what we need when we need it. What you have and who you are are enough for you to be called " divine goddess."

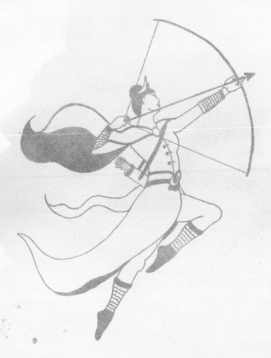

Lady Xian, Chinese goddess of protection

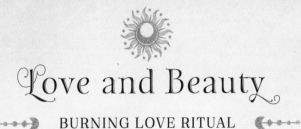

Love and Beauty

BURNING LOVE RITUAL

When you need to fan the dying embers in a relationship to benefit from its warming heat, slip into a warm bath scattered with rose petals—placing some under your pillow can help, too.

GATHER:

Red candle

Sturdy, heatproof surface

Rose quartz crystals or garnets, for love

Matches

15 drops rose essential oil mixed with
1 tablespoon (15 ml) carrier oil, such as almond, jojoba, or olive

Rose petals or a rose

1. Fill your tub with soothing warm water.

2. Place the candle on the sturdy surface. Place the crystals around the candle to cast your circle. Light the candle.

3. Pour the essential oil mix into the tub and swirl it around with your hand to distribute. Be aware of the sensation of the water—feel the fluid caress and softness.

4. Scatter the rose petals onto the water's surface and let their loving symbolism infuse the water. Imagine the water is about to embrace you like a lover.

5. Slip into the bath and relax into the sensual feel of the water. Gaze softly into the candle's flame as you feel your energy rise. Take a moment in silent gratitude for the life-giving water and opportunity for self-care.

6. Invite your goddess into your circle. Close your eyes and, when ready, say quietly or aloud:

*Such beauty as yours ignites flames of desire. I seek to touch
your soul with mine to light my flame within.*

*Venus [or goddess of choice], grant me your smoldering
passion that burns without end to excite.*

*A lesson in charm meant to tempt without
harm can transform me as day into night.*

*With petals as soft as my lover's sweet kiss,
I place roses as thanks at your feet.*

*In fire as bright as your burning delight,
I see my lover awaiting tonight.*

Be cautious when stepping out of the tub; it may be slippery.

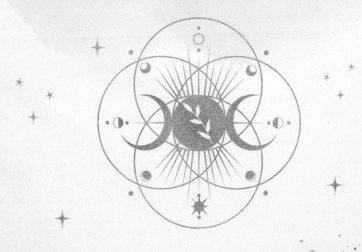

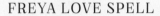 ## FREYA LOVE SPELL

That passionate type of adoring love that leaves you feeling you can tackle anything is a magic all its own. When your desire is to ignite the flame and turn up the heat in your life, numerous love goddesses will be there to cheer you on—Freya will be chief among them.

With runes dispersed and fates held tight,
I turn to Freya's magic sight.

Reveal when love will come my way,
when passion burns without delay.

Among the secrets of your charms,
your beauty is like a siren's call.

Teach me the tempting chant to haunt
the dreams of lovers I do want.

FINDING A MATCH!

There is no shortage of goddess allies to offer opinions and advice on attracting the perfect mate. If that's what's on your mind, pour some wine (or tea, or other favorite beverage—one for you, one for your goddess BFF) and settle in for a chat. You can meditate on who may be the one, journal with your goddess on taking the first step, sit outside and listen to the sounds of the Universe for cues that say the timing is right . . . whatever appeals to you. When ready, say quietly or aloud:

*Bewitch me with your graceful charms and
cast a spell that does no harm.*

*For love is what my heart desires
and has in sight a fond admirer.*

*Do help me make my message clear:
I wish to bring our lips so near*

*that searing heat does melt our fears and
happily we'll live for years.*

GODDESS BEAUTY QUEEN

Goddess, goddess, loved by all, who's the fairest one of all? Most say Aphrodite, but today, it's you! Loving yourself unconditionally must happen first before anyone else can fully love you the way you want to be loved. And there's no harm in having a little fun to beautify that self-love. Dress up in some fancy clothes, layer on the bling, a little make-up, if you please, and get ready to accept the crown from the original "beauty queen," Aphrodite—who may also lend a little sex appeal to the occasion. So, make some plans to be adored. When ready to be crowned Goddess Beauty Queen, say quietly or aloud:

Fairest goddess, loved by all, born rising from the sea,

to gaze at you is but pure bliss; your beauty is my plea:

Do place your crown upon my head that gorgeous I may be.

O queen of love and grace divine, please tell me what you see.

A goddess true whose beauty shines without apology,

adored by all, but best of all, herself unconditionally.

AURA OF ENCHANTMENT

To make yourself irresistible to that certain someone, send out an aura of enchantment. Let yourself exude mystery, allure, and spellbinding beauty. Call your goddess allies to channel their enchanting ways. Ask The Muses to accompany you as you say quietly or aloud to your certain someone:

*With face to tempt and words to woo,
enchantment has its eyes on you.*

*For in my spell you will remain, enraptured
so with love's refrain.*

*This goddess aura flows from me
and binds us for eternity.*

*Resist no more my true desire—
surrender to love's growing fire.*

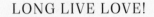 ## LONG LIVE LOVE!

When you find that special someone, love seems so easy. As it ages, though, it does take more work to keep it alive. It ebbs and flows and changes and grows, just like the seasons. Learning to go with the flow is key to making love last. It is something to be worshipped and celebrated in its own right. Take wisdom from any goddess of love you trust and say quietly or aloud, as often as you like, to conjure a lifetime of love that holds up to anything:

When love chooses you, all the world seems anew.
Dear goddess, please grant me this wish:

May what's new today weather well and
turn gray as the fires of passion do die,

but smoldering still have the heat to sustain
through both good times and darkness of night.

When life's reached its end, my prayer is that, then,
our love still shines blindingly bright.

Marriage, Fertility, and Motherhood

EARTH MOTHER HARVEST DINNER

What could be more worthy of celebration than the mothers that birth us, the harvest that feeds us, the wisdom that nurtures us, and the love that sustains us? Put your magical cauldron to work creating a feast to honor all Mother Goddesses everywhere with a special Earth Mother Harvest Dinner. Whatever time of year or occasion you choose to celebrate with this special ritual, try to incorporate meaningful foods based on your intentions, and honor those dear to you who have passed by including their favorite foods.

The reasons to gather likeminded friends and family are many: to name a few, new pregnancies and births (think: baby showers), the glorious colors of spring's rebirth, celebrations of the wisdom of mothers everywhere, the ripe bounty of summer, the first harvest that will feed us through leaner times, even the time to savor the stillness that lays the groundwork for future harvests. Add your favorite reason to celebrate the bounty that Earth Mothers produce, the bounty that breathes life into us in so many ways.

Because every food has magical properties, deciding which to include is a purely personal choice! Prepare the food with respect and honor, imbuing it with your wishes and intentions. Be mindful of the outcomes you desire and stir joy and gratitude into every spoonful.

SAMPLE HARVEST MENU

Apples, avocados, eggs, milk, and pomegranates for fertility and love

Barley, beets, corn, and potatoes to celebrate Earth Mother Goddesses all

Bread and beer to honor the grain harvest and goddess Ceres

Cakes to honor the sweet sacrifices all mothers make

Chocolate and strawberries for love and romance

Cinnamon for abundance

Coriander, garlic, honey, marjoram, mint, and thyme for health

Cornmeal for celebrating the harvest

Grapes for garden magic

Olives for peace

Oranges as a symbol of the life-nurturing Sun

Peach and sage for wisdom

Rice for rain to feed the crops

Rosemary for remembrance of loved ones passed

Sesame, sunflower, and poppy seeds for growth and opportunity

Wine for bounty and celebration

May the gathering here be a visible homage to the
Earth Mother Goddess, creator of all life.

May the foods offered here nurture
bodies, health, and desires.

May the drink offered here celebrate the bounty
of life and the joy of the living.

May the gratitude we show with respect to the Earth
honor the goddess in us all.

May the Earth Mother Goddess be pleased and
bestow blessings in return.

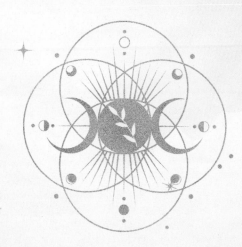

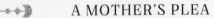 A MOTHER'S PLEA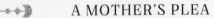

The birth of a new baby is one of life's magical miracles. Turn to any Mother Goddess or goddess of fertility whose energy matches yours to infuse your world with fertile possibilities.

O Mother Goddess, hear my plea
and turn your fertile gaze on me.

The time is ripe, I truly feel—
for deep within a stir I feel

that rocks me to my core with love and
yearns to hold, from stars above,

a babe born unto life with me—
to nurture, grow, and then set free.

For love to change the world is born
each time you fill a mother's arms.

A MOTHER'S EMBRACE

Danu, mother of all Irish gods and people, including the fairy people, brings us the comfort, love, and acceptance of a mother. As goddess of water, love flows from her like an endless river. She surely has generations of experience giving those hugs that mothers are so famous for! Turn to her when you're in need of a reassuring embrace in today's tumultuous world. When ready, say quietly or aloud, Great mother Danu:

In every ripple of a pond, in every twinkle of the sea, I feel your presence next to me.

Envelop me within your arms that I may float there safe from harm.

Your soothing love flows into me, embraced through all eternity.

VOW OF COMMITMENT

Goddesses with the most successful unions stay true to themselves while also committing to the good of the team. If commitment is in your future, turn to your favorite goddess for advice on living your true self in a way that benefits you and your partner.

O Goddess Realm of unions blessed,
please turn your thoughts my way.

Commitment comes in many forms
and with your help I pray,

that giving love and keeping vows
are sacred in their ways,

of joining two, then, into one, while each still has a say.

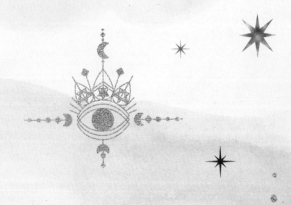

PACHAMAMA GROUNDING EXERCISE

Evoke Pachamama, ultimate Earth Mother, when a bit of grounding is in order. Grounding can be a way for you to release excess energy as well as to draw energy from the Earth. It can help you feel safe, calm, and centered, to keeping you in the present moment when stress and worry threaten to get in the way of manifesting your goals. It's simple:

1. Step outside barefoot—walk in the grass, lie in the sand, dip your toes in a lake—to physically connect with the energies of the Earth.

2. To release excess energy: Press down into the Earth with your legs and feet; even place your hands on the ground and press, if you like. Visualize the energy you need to release moving into the Earth as she absorbs it and spreads it away from you.

3. To draw energy: Stand, sit, or lie on the ground. Close your eyes if you are comfortable, and imagine the Earth's electrical charge filling you, charging your batteries. Lie there until you feel fully replenished.

4. When ready, say quietly or aloud:

Pachamama, Mother Goddess,
stand with me in connection to Earth.

Walk gently by my side that my footsteps do no harm
as I send my energies deep into Earth's heart.

Lie beside me as I feel Earth fill me
with vibrations from her core.

Take my hand that we are one with Earth,
in this moment, at ease and at peace.

Blessed be.

FAMILY BLESSINGS

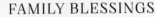

Mother Goddesses know that families come in many forms and grow and change over time. Honor the common thread among all: love. Appeal to your favorite matriarch goddess for her guidance and blessings to keep watch over your family. When ready, say quietly or aloud:

Dear Mother Goddess of unending love, I thank you for the family you have sent me from above.

Grant me wisdom in tending their needs that stronger our bonds may grow.

Guide me with grace to celebrate our differences as well as our common strengths.

Give me the courage to weather the worries that inevitably I must face.

Teach me to see when each branch of our tree has blossomed and grown on its own.

Open my heart to your loving embrace so that there is room for the family to grow.

Bless us, each one, with the freedom that comes from a love that gives flight to our dreams.

Relationships, Truth, and Forgiveness

When working with a group to amplify energies feels like the right choice, gather your friends to mark a specific goddess celebration or for any occasion to connect, celebrate, and amplify manifesting energies in a goddess circle. The purpose of your circle is to celebrate and honor the goddess and all her gifts, to open yourself to her power, increasing energy, intuition, and goddess wisdom.

Your circle is your sacred space to work your magic. Cast it with physical objects, such as crystals, candles (safely), stones, fruit, strewing herbs or flowers; sprinkle eco-friendly glitter outside; or simply draw it in the air with your finger. Casting is simply connecting with the energies of the Earth and Universe. It is a place to gather and a place to create and release goddess energy. It is a haven of learning, sharing, meditating, and lifting others up. It is a powerful place to work with the Goddess Realm.

1. Invite your friends to step inside the circle to connect and amplify their energies by joining hands, standing or sitting, around an altar, if you wish.

2. If you like, each person can place an object representing their goddess, or an offering to their goddess, or representing their intentions for the ceremony inside the circle or on the altar.

3. Invite the goddesses to join you in the circle.

4. Use the circle for intention setting or to draw the goddesses' abundant energies to you. Create and chant your own mantra to raise the energies around you. Stand or sit silently in meditation on your intentions. Sing, walk, or dance clockwise in the circle. Why clockwise? The spinning clockwise energy brings things to you. Share intentions aloud, or offer them quietly to the Universe.

5. As offerings of food and drink are welcome goddess favors, consider a simple toast to the goddess and light snacks to pass in the circle as a sign of gratitude for the many gifts the goddess brings.

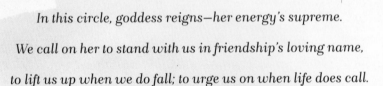

In this circle, goddess reigns—her energy's supreme.

We call on her to stand with us in friendship's loving name,

to lift us up when we do fall; to urge us on when life does call.

With wine and food we honor her
and walk her path in gratitude

for lessons learned and strength renewed.

6. To close the circle, light a candle in memory of someone unable to be there and take a moment to give thanks for the blessings they brought to your life. Take a moment to give thanks for the many blessings bestowed by your chosen goddess and the blessing of friends. Walk or dance counterclockwise, which dispels or banishes the energy, to dissolve the circle. *Blessed be.*

GODDESS TEA

When your inner goddess needs a reboot, it's time for goddess tea. While a tea ceremony can be an elaborate ritual (and one you may want to devote to a goddess someday), all you need here are two cups of hot tea: one for you, one for your goddess—and a bit of time to fortify your relationship with yourself. Perhaps hibiscus to honor your delicate beauty, jasmine to ignite your sensuality, lavender for calm and renewal, chamomile for rest, lemon for joy, rosehips for creativity, or Saint-John's-wort for courage. Invite the appropriate goddess to join you and offer a cup of tea in gratitude.

To increase the intimacy, offer a tea from your goddess's country of origin, or one made from her sacred herbs, or with Moon water for its special energy. Sit someplace quiet and undisturbed, inhale the aromas, and savor the flavors and energies in the cup while meditating on your issue at hand. When ready, say quietly or aloud:

I've brewed this tea, cast this spell,
and conjured goddess energy.

Recharge my soul, refill my cup,
with your wings do lift me up

Goddess-charged my life may be
and linked with you eternally.

With goddess grace, your help I pray;
with goddess courage I seize the day.

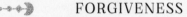

FORGIVENESS

All relationships, in order to thrive, require forgiving and forgiveness.
No matter whether you are giving or receiving, you must do so from a
true heart. Forgiveness releases pain and makes room for love to grow.
With help from your favorite goddess, say quietly or aloud:

*O goddess whose grace is forgiveness
and whose forgiveness is grace, walk with me.*

*Forgiveness is hard, whether earned on my own,
or given to others in need.*

*Show me the path that leads to the well of
those healing waters you speak of,*

*for there I can drink of the balm that will lead
to the soothing forgiveness I seek.*

TRUTH TELLING

We're all tempted to tell those little white lies—what's the harm? Well, one lie is never enough, and pretty soon, you can't tell fact from fiction. Plus, no one likes being lied to. Stick to the truth. It's the right thing to do. Call on your trusted truth allies when times do tempt.

Goddess of truth, hear my plea, that fooled by lies I never be;

that when I'm tempted not to say what's in my heart, you'll call to me,

a warning that, fooled not you'll be, but lies do make a fool of thee.

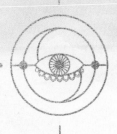

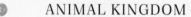 ## ANIMAL KINGDOM

Many goddesses have faithful animal companions ever by their side to love them, protect them, adorn them, transport them, amuse them, and more! To ensure your beloved animal companions stay healthy, safe, and happy, evoke any goddess who shares your animal passion. When ready, say quietly or aloud:

A prayer for all the animals, upon the Earth who roam,

their gentle love, a gift so pure,
there's none that can compare.

Please bless my sweet companions
for their ever-faithful ways—

an endless well of love that pours each
day from doting eyes.

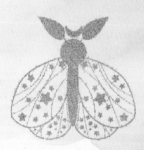

GIVE LOVE—ALWAYS

I particularly like Amaterasu and Kuan Yin for this reminder: Do not withhold love—ever. When important relationships leave us feeling hurt or let down, it's easy to withdraw and withhold love as punishment. You're only punishing yourself and hurting those who love you in the process. While not always easy, remember, love begets love with its tender care. Speak to Amaterasu for help seeing the truth in this, and Kuan Yin for compassionate wisdom when pain or anger threatens to draw you inward.

When love does falter, lights go dim and spirits cease to dance.
I call for goddess help to lift me from this aching trance.

With humble grace to you, I pray to guide me to the light; to
warm my soul with loving words that quell the urge to fight.

To open wide my eyes to see that love is always right.

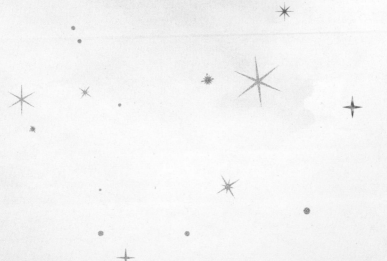

GIVE AND TAKE

Relationships thrive when each person involved is allowed to be an individual as well as a member of the team. Managing conflicting expectations requires a give and take, and the flexibility that acceptance and nonjudgment afford. Call on any of the Mother Goddesses for their spirit of unconditional love to help when the relationship road feels a little rocky, or the love goddesses to remind you why you're in the relationship in the first place! When ready, say quietly or aloud:

O goddesses who love so true, hear my fervent plea:

Fill me with your patient love that
ne'er complains nor favors me,

but watches as the bloom unfolds
with loving mind and heart of gold.

Each seed will have its chance to grow,
to face the Sun, to feel its time.

This timeless dance of trading leads,
gives time to rest and time to breathe.

Home, Hearth, and Healing

THE MAGIC OF MUSIC

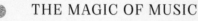

Music—from The Muses—can fill a home with its magic. Music's vibrations affect our vibrations and can help clear emotional and physical blockages so that positive energy flows freely once again. A music-filled home inspires physical movement, reduces stress, relaxes the body, promotes better sleep, eases depression, boosts verbal intelligence in children, and keeps our brains active—all components of magical goddess living. Invite The Muses to your next dance party, or evoke any goddess whose magical energies will bless your home and all who dwell within.

Sweet music of The Muses,
fill my home with joy.

Where music dwells so beauty lives and
blessings freely flow.

Each note a blooming flower with
its messages of hope;

my hearth becomes a home
where music's healing fills the soul.

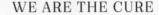

With all the suffering the world has recently undergone, it's easy to feel overwhelmed and underprepared to make a difference. Remember, every change begins with one small action, and one small action of kindness aimed at another, whose burden we cannot know, will ease our burden threefold.

The goddess Panacea was said to have a poultice with which she healed all. As an alternative, I suggest calling on your goddess healers, and especially Panacea, to summon their poultice wisdom and send its healing energies out into the Universe. You may want to diffuse a soothing essential oil, such as lavender or pine, to set the mood. When ready to lend healing vibrations to your world or the world at large, say quietly or aloud:

*Where silent ills do spread their fear
and keep us far from those held dear,*

*the healing Sun must spread its rays,
diffuse the clouds, infuse the day*

*with hope that cure for which we pray
does usher in recovery's way.*

*O goddess, with your healing might,
do spread your wings and soothe our plight.*

*Uplift our souls with soothing balm,
deliver us from all that harms.*

Whether physical, emotional, or spiritual, healing is a process. Summon your inner goddess strength and sit with any goddess of healing that resonates with you. Airmid is a favorite for her vast herbal healing knowledge and compassion.

Gather a black candle for protection or a green candle to channel the herbs Airmid works with, an amethyst or clear quartz crystal for its healing energies, and any healing herbs you can, such as angelica, bay leaf, fennel, ivy, lemon balm, or marigold. Essential oils can stand in—try chamomile, lavender, rose, sandalwood, or peppermint.

Dress the candle with essential oil if you wish. Light the candle. Muddle or crush the fresh herbs in your cauldron, if you have one, to release their healing oils, aromas, and energies. Take a deep breath in and hold it, letting the herbal energies and the life-sustaining oxygen reach deep throughout your body. Exhale slowly. Continue to breathe this way, focusing your breath and its healing energies on the part of your body that you wish to heal, including your mind, heart, or soul. When ready, say quietly or aloud:

That which heals can also harm,
respect I must these herbal balms.

With thoughts attuned to easing pain,
I pray your healing hands to lay

upon my [area to be healed],
draw ills away and speed release, to mend I may.

The body may be first to feel but mind
and heart are next to heal.

With time, as wounds do fade away,
I'll not forget your help this day.

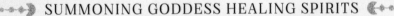
When you or someone you love is ailing, turn to any goddess of healing for this ritual. Best outcomes for rituals like this happen when working on your own behalf, but when no harm is intended, only healing, you may also perform this on behalf of others. Consider their circumstances and wishes before doing so.

On your altar or working in your sacred space, gather:

Almonds, as an offering to invoke the healing powers of the goddess chosen

Small glass of pure water

Goddess statue or picture, if you like

1 blue (calming energy) or red (warming energy) candle for healing

Matches

Paper

Pen

Cauldron

1. Place the almonds and water on your altar next to the goddess statue, if you have one, as an offering.

2. Light the candle, whose energy will help release your prayer into the world. Take a moment in silent meditation to call forth the goddess whose healing powers you seek. Visualize her with you. Acknowledge her presence.

3. On your paper, write down the specific illness and symptoms that you wish to be relieved, as well as what you desire to replace them. Fold the paper as small as you can and place it into the cauldron on a heatproof surface.

4. Pray to your goddess for healing relief:

O goddess [name], I feel your healing spirit. Place your curing
touch upon [name] to dispel the ills that grip.

With water from your sacred font,
do purify the wounds you see and those that hide inside.

Bring peaceful thoughts to ease
the fear and help to calm the dread.

With breath of life do sing of times
when health and joy resume.

Please banish pain and restore
strength that healing does ensue.

For this we honor you, give thanks, for what we ask of you.

5. Take a moment to sit in gratitude for what the goddess will bring.

6. Light the paper in your cauldron and watch the flames carry away
    the illness and pain you wish to be eased. Carefully extinguish the
    flames with the water, as needed.

7. Extinguish the candle and watch the rising smoke take your
    prayer into the cosmos, where it will be received and answered.

SLEEP LIKE A GODDESS

When sleeping like an angel proves a devil of a fight, evoke any goddess of the night or one who can bring sleep with a soft touch of her hand. Get comfortable, breathe in the sweet scent of stardust, and speak to your chosen goddess. When ready, say quietly or aloud:

O lovely goddess, sleep I seek wrapped gently in your wings.

Do whisper soothing words of calm,
like angels when they sing.

The peace I seek lies in sweet rest, sublime above all things.

Please ease these restless nights I fear,
deep sleep I pray you'll bring.

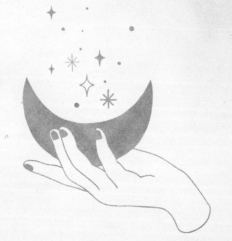

Abundance, Good Fortune, and Prosperity

CLEAR NEGATIVE ENERGY

Sometimes, what seems like a run of bad luck or misfortune is really just the need to become unstuck. Cleansing our psyches can clear the effects of accumulated negative energies that may be holding us back. Evoke any goddess you connect with, whose energies offer cleansing, flowing, abundant powers, or any Moon goddess who can join you at the height of the Full Moon, when her purifying energy is at its highest, to cleanse, restore, and celebrate the ritual of making room for new, positive energies to fill you.

Carrying or wearing crystals whose energies are in tune with your intentions can also be helpful. Consider black tourmaline or selenite (banishing negative energy), rose quartz (filling you with unconditional love, compassion, peace), clear quartz (all-purpose cleansing power), moonstone, of course (connecting to your inner goddess), or amethyst (protection).

Call on your goddess and sit with her in meditation. Breathe. Deeply in. Slowly out. Again. Focus your thoughts on filling your body with the goddess's flowing vitality on every breath in. Let yourself feel it travel throughout your body. Breathe out any negativity still blocking the way to an abundant, prosperous life. Stay with your goddess as long as is comfortable and gently retune to the world around you when finished, then say to your goddess quietly or aloud:

As air flows in and feeds my lungs
your love flows in to feed the soul.

Each breath replaces dark with light that flows
through me with cleansing might—

the rhythm of my life's restored,
with humble thanks, you are adored.

181

FEELIN' LUCKY

Hope and luck go hand in hand, but why not increase the odds by dealing in your favorite fortune goddess. She's got your back. A generous offering could seal the deal.

When the Moon shines bright
and my luck feels right, it's the perfect time to bet

that my blessings came—Lady Luck's her name—
as an answer to my plea.

Sweet goddess, cast your spell for me—
set kismet, karma, fortune free

to boost the probability your Wheel of Fortune favors me.

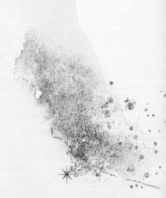

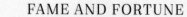 ## FAME AND FORTUNE

We're all destined for our fifteen minutes of goddess fame, but some of us just want more. When you crave the spotlight, and plan to use it for good, ask your favorite goddess to shine her beacon on you. Carrying a lucky penny, sprig of dill, and piece of jade will amplify your message. Don't be afraid to grab the mic when it's presented to make your message known. When you're ready for your close-up, say quietly or aloud:

With goddess poise and goddess pose,
envisioned riches thus bestowed,

and endless days spent pampered so
that I don't need to lift a toe

with all my wants supremely met—
arrived at last, my life's the best.

But something more inside me calls
to spread the wealth and so the cause:

Each life is famous for its worth,
defined by joy each day from birth.

SWEET SUCCESS

Lakshmi, ultimate goddess of wealth and success, may be just the one to call upon when cash reserves are dwindling, but the spirit to earn more burns bright. When ready, say quietly or aloud:

Sweet Lakshmi, of whose beauty sings
of joy and wealth and all she brings.

Upon your lotus throne you sit:
my prayer is that you move a bit . . .

that I may join you on the seat whose
symbol tells of wealth so sweet.

Please heed my prayer, that so endowed,
my life is rich with your bequeath.

ABUNDANT WISHES

A generous spirit is the foundation of abundance. Giving is receiving and receiving is born of gratitude. The Goddess Realm is filled with generosity, blessed with plenty, and eager to support you in living an abundant life. Set your intentions accordingly and walk with your chosen goddess toward your destination. When ready to begin, say quietly or aloud:

> *With steps unsure I take your hand—*
> *to follow in your footsteps grand.*
>
> *My grateful heart is full of plans,*
> *like seeds to plant in fertile land.*
>
> *Guide me along this winding path;*
> *teach me to cull the wheat from chaff,*
>
> *that blessed with bounty I may*
> *be to share with all humanity.*

Wisdom and Knowledge

This simple meditation ritual can help you appeal to the ancient Moon goddesses who came before you. Their wisdom and guidance in these changing and emotional times are available to you simply by asking.

Each goddess can awaken different sacred feminine aspects within, so feel free to ask for all their gifts, or a specific one, depending on your needs. Connecting is simple:

1. Sit in quiet meditation (see page 17) and concentrate on the goddess you wish to invite in and any specific area you wish to work on with her. For example, invite Isis to boost your confidence and intuition to tackle a specific situation. When meditating, connect with the goddesses in whatever way resonates with you.

2. There's nothing more to it than inviting her in and sitting quietly in meditation. Pay attention to your intuitive senses: *clairaudience* (clear healing), *clairsentience* (clear feeling), *claircognizance* (clear knowing), and *clairvoyance* (clear seeing). Depending on which sense is strongest, you may hear, feel, know, or see her guidance, presence, and love.

3. No matter what, trust that by simply asking for the goddesses' support you open yourself to connect with your divine feminine gifts, which reveal themselves subtly and mysteriously. Be alert for signs of their guidance and trust your intuition when working with the goddesses.

4. Offer thanks to your goddess for her time and attention.

There are those times when the facts alone just don't provide enough information, times when the wisdom and knowledge of what to do—or not do—meanmean the difference between success and failure. Understanding the hidden implications of the messages we receive, and acting on them appropriately, sometimes means calling on a higher—goddess—power. When those moments face you, offer the following (quietly or aloud) to the wise goddess you choose, and be open to her illuminating messages:

O knowing goddess, lend your help
for sagely must I see,

my head says, "Yes," my heart says,
"No"—my friends, not one agrees.

With choices hard, and outcomes real,
please wisely advise me.

KITCHEN WISDOM

We spend a lot of time in the kitchen preparing food to nourish ourselves, our friends, and our families. Stir your cauldron wisely and with intention to infuse your meals with the wisdom you wish to impart. Call on a combination of hearth and wise goddesses, especially Cerridwen, to lend recipes to your collection. Once you've established your intentions, say quietly or aloud:

A sprig of basil lends great courage
when rocky roads prevail.

A frond of dill, a sprig of mint—
keep safe along life's trail.

A pinch of sage for in those times
when wisdom it does fail,

and yarrow leaves to heal what
hurts and comfort what does ail.

Some cinnamon, when sprinkled on,
smells sweetly of success,

with lavender and chamomile
for sleep and peaceful rest.

So, stir and sip and add a dash
of salt for flavor's sake—

my wish for you, a seasoned life,
is there for you to take.

TRY A NEW PERSPECTIVE

The wisest goddesses among us know there is much to learn from others. Different perspectives can open whole realms of unseen possibilities. To challenge your own perspective, swap chairs at dinner, take a different seat in a business meeting, sit facing the opposite direction on the subway . . . a simple change can spark a new outlook. When ready to challenge your perspective, call on those goddesses you love whose roles seem quite contradictory, and say quietly or aloud:

*O goddess whose role seems to differ
as much as by night and by day,*

*Do teach me your unspoken wisdom
to take in all life has to say . . .*

*for stuck in a rut I can be, with thoughts
all turned inward on me.*

*But widen my angle I must, to ensure
my actions breed trust,*

*and help me remember to say,
thank you for sharing your way.*

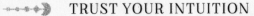 **TRUST YOUR INTUITION**

Your intuition is the well of wisdom that accumulates in your gut over a lifetime of experience. It is your goddess power to assess the unseen and know when there's danger ahead. It sees clearly, even when we don't, which is why we tend to second-guess it. Many goddesses are attuned to their subconscious's ability to see what we ignore. Iris, as one, can be evoked when head and heart do not align.

All-seeing goddess whose presence I seek,
grant me the power to see.

I call on you to heed my cry, awaken sights within.
Power my internal eye, make clear what I deny.

LETTING GO

The beauty of releasing something that no longer serves is in the freedom it provides—from guilt, from worry, from fear, from disappointment. In its place is a wide-open space ready to be filled with intentions that align with our priorities. Crone goddesses, particularly Hecate, can help us see clearly when that time has come. When ready to face the reality, say quietly or aloud:

Goddess of darkness, whose wisdom is light,
whose knowledge increases with time,

an ending is but a beginning, you teach,
to shed what no longer is mine.

Please grant me the grace to freely let go
of what does not serve and what does not grow.

To see there's a path that invites me to climb,
away from the past and step toward the sublime.

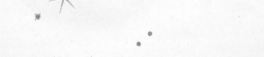

Strength and Protection

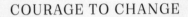
Sometimes, bad habits can keep us from reaching our goals, and frequently undermine our true intentions. What holds us back is often the fear of change. When the time is right to commit to a change, you may have to commit to defeating the behavior getting in your way. Acknowledge the goddess you call to your side, and take a few moments to visualize *your* goddess courage, feeling the strength of commitment. When ready, say quietly or aloud:

Good goddess, join this fearsome
fight to keep my worthy goals in sight.
Grant courage that habits rued this day,
in battle fall and fade away.

To conquer fear that holds me back,
commit to change I must attack.

Thus, armed am I to see this through,
each hope and dream achieving true.

STRENGTH TO PERSEVERE

As we battle through our everyday lives, it's easy to lose sight of what's important. The endless rush, noise, and chaos can drown out our thoughts and leave little time for manifesting intentions. Call on the warrior goddesses to help settle your conflicts and protect your time and space so you can persevere in the work that brings inner peace. Athena is a perfect ally. When ready, say quietly or aloud:

Athena, born dressed for battle—
warrior right from the start.

Grant me the courage to mark and
defend the boundaries true to my heart.

Instill in me strength to persevere, too,
in facing the fight to the end.

For there I will find the peace that I seek,
with olive branch firmly in hand.

PANTHEON OF PROTECTION

In these challenging times, when we often feel pushed to the brink by unseen harm everywhere we turn, it's easy to feel scared and uncertain. Separated from loved ones and what was our everyday life, we crave a need for the familiar. As we move toward healing, call on your goddess allies to multiply their protective energies to keep you safe while navigating the path forward.

I call on the pantheon of goddesses here—
join hands, raise energies for good.

For evil roams the world,
forsaking not a neighborhood.

Fight we must, to rid our homes
from harm we cannot see.

Do cast your goddess strength as shield,
protecting all—blessed be.

GUARDIAN GODDESS PRAYER

When we know what's right but feel unprepared for the fight, a goddess whose influence includes strength, truth, and power can be our best ally. Don't be afraid to ask for help.

In times of darkness, bring your light.
In times of fear, clear my sight.

Mighty goddess, stand with me
to give me courage to fight the fight.

For peace I pray and strength to stand
for what is right, which will demand

a courage so deep I fear I'll fail,
but with your help I will prevail.

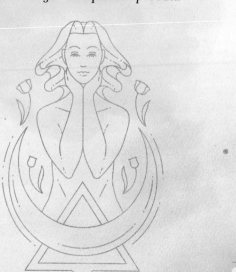

STRENGTH TO BELIEVE IN MAGIC

Each goddess of the Goddess Realm brings her special gifts to the world—chief among them: magic. The magic to believe—in her powers, her fate, love, the unseen, the unproven—in her magic. Living with strength to believe in magic gives us the gift of magic in belief. Gather your magical goddess friends, and say quietly or aloud:

In sunsets, stars, and rainbows, too,
the magic of the world shines through.

Though magic isn't always seen,
but felt inside—a joy that's keen.

I cherish every kiss I thought was
goddess wings, a fairy's taunt.

The trail of blessings left behind
is magic of a special kind . . .

When searching for the magic true,
just look inside: It's there in you.

Creativity and Joy

Living joyfully is defined by you. Take a moment to think about what brings you true joy, then commit to making it a priority. Living joyfully also means living in the moment—no time for regret and no chance to worry about the future. See all that you have and be grateful for what fills your world. Leave judgment by the wayside and accept all the joy life brings. Seek goddess joy in all you do and let it shine forth from your smile. Working with your favorite goddess of happiness, say quietly or aloud:

O goddess of pure heart and mind,
whose joyful presence brings delight.

Do teach me of your song and dance—
their merriment is like a trance

that settles deep within my soul,
transforming darkness into light.

Each smile, breath, and movement, too,
speaks gaiety in laughing hues,

to color life with gleeful mirth that blesses
each new day with worth.

CELEBRATE YOUR INNER GODDESS EACH DAY

Every day brings with it goddess possibilities for embracing who you are. Don't waste another day diminishing your goddess aura. Let it shine into the world—its energy will create its own magic.

Mirror, mirror, talk to me:
Describe the goddess that you see.

"O goddess standing there in sight,
I see within a mighty might.

Your face a beam of Moonlight glow;
your eyes spill love your heart does know.

You nurture, teach, and create life—
you fight the fight and ease the strife.

Your goddess wisdom guides us all;
your graceful gifts do grace us all."

Believe in goddess power true—
each goddess sees herself in you.

UNLEASH YOUR GODDESS CREATIVITY

Creative moods can strike anywhere, anytime—but sometimes they need a little nudge to reveal themselves. In addition to calling on any goddess who inspires you with her passion, or a particular goddess associated with an art or craft, incorporating crystals into your goddess magic can lend an energetic boost to the creative equation. Try citrine for pure creativity; blue lace agate to align your head and heart; amethyst or another purple crystal for expanded imagination; carnelian for unleashing creative thoughts; celestite for divine inspiration; or opal for truest self-expression. Holding your crystal and feeling your goddess guiding you, when ready, say quietly or aloud:

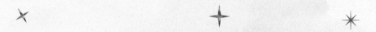

In humble awe of who you are, of all that you create,

do breathe new life into my soul, do help me celebrate

the passion that I know can find a way to show the world

the magic of my art within—my story yet untold.

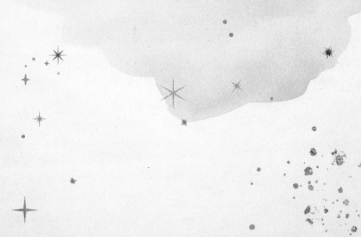

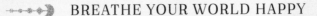
Just the faintest glimpse of a rainbow can instill in us with immeasurable joy—and signal a message from the divine. Although not rare, they do not come around every day . . . so use their imagery to conjure happiness anytime you need a mood lift or adjustment. Red, orange, yellow, green, blue, indigo, and violet are the colors that paint the bridge in the sky and dissolve into our minds with their energies.

Before you begin, call on Iris, goddess of the rainbow, to inspire joyful mantras to vibrate within and open your heart and mind to all the happiness around you. When ready, say quietly or aloud:

Breathe and believe: I am joy, I am light, I am peace.

Breathe and believe: I am strong, I am here, I am enough.

Breathe and believe: I have hope, I have love, I have all.

Find a peaceful, quiet location. Close your eyes, if you are comfortable doing so, and breathe in each color, one at a time, letting it fill you from head to toe as it instills in you with its vitality and joy.

- Red: Breathe in passion; breathe out pain.

- Orange: Breathe in creativity; breathe out boredom.

- Yellow: Breathe in the joyful, life-giving qualities of the Sun; breathe out fear.

- Green: Breathe in renewal; breathe out sorrow.

- Blue: Breathe in calm; breathe out tension.

- Indigo: Breathe in intuition; breathe out negativity.

- Violet: Breathe in messages from your goddess; breathe out gratitude.

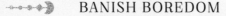 BANISH BOREDOM

Boredom and routine can sap creativity and joy. Infuse a little goddess creativity into your world with an essential oil and your favorite creative deity, such as The Muses, to help ignite the spark. Lovely scents were sacred to the goddesses and used in numerous ceremonies and rites, so they'll be at home on your altar when you need an extra something to dispel the negative energies that boredom breeds. Citrus scents are fresh and just the thing to add a little "zest" to your day.

Gentle Muse, whose talent does
amuse and bring delight,

on feather breeze, soft through the trees,
enchant my world tonight.

Guide my hand to paint my days
in colors bold and bright;

infuse my soul with lyric glow,
turning darkness into light.

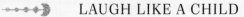 ## LAUGH LIKE A CHILD

Remember those silly jokes that made you laugh 'til you cried as a kid—or now cause your kids to break into hysterics? Remember how good it felt? A good belly laugh not only breathes fun into your day but also literally causes you to breathe good oxygen into your body, stimulates circulation, eases muscle tension, boosts your mood, connects you to others, eases stress and pain, and activates your immune system. That is something to laugh about! The goddess Baubo has one of the bawdiest senses of humor in the goddess kingdom. She is sure to induce at least a giggle, if not a chuckle, and hopefully a full-on fit of laughter. When ready to laugh yourself healthy, say quietly or aloud:

Dear Baubo, mistress of great fun,
your talents are required:

Please shimmy, jiggle, dance,
and prance to your heart's desire.

A joke or two thrown in the mix
will please the crowd, no doubt,

for full-on mirth and laughter's birth,
we pray, you will inspire.

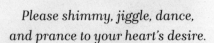
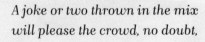

Well, charmed I am, and blessed to spend abundant time with you.
Each goddess friend shows us again how strength has many hues.

We've tackled love and family, home and health, and wisdom, too.
We've laughed and cried, and wondered how on Earth we've muddled through.

Forgiveness now comes easier, as we know it's born of love,
And beauty is as beauty does—alluring its admirers!

Creative juices flow when in the company of others—
We've even talked about the day we turned into our mothers!

This time, well spent, with just "the girls" has given me a gift—
The chance to be myself among the greatest who uplift.

Thank you, Goddess Realm, for opening your circle wide to me,
Your wisdom, love, and guidance helped me see who I could be.

As pages close, it's not the end of friendships old or new,
For here we've built foundations strong—the rest is up to you.

Acknowledgments

As with a child, it takes a goddess village to raise a book. Thanks first to my goddess-like editor, Leeann Moreau. Your faith in me, as well as your words of encouragement, inspiration, strategy, and compassion, were your goddess gifts to me during the writing of this book. And as always, chief goddess and publisher, Rage Kindelsperger, led with wisdom and authority. Special thanks are due, too, to the rest of the team at Wellfleet, gods and goddesses alike, for lending their immense talents to this creative endeavor.

To my family and friends: Thank you for your support, enthusiasm, interest, and encouragement. They are blessings and a joy. To my sister-goddess, Gaye, I honor your strength. To my husband, John: Your unwavering love and support and worship of my goddess status in the home are gifts from the gods!

To my readers, gods and goddesses all, thank you. Blessed be.

Resources and References

Akta Lakota Museum and Cultural Center. "Legend of the White Buffalo." AktaLakota.stjo.org. Accessed April 6, 2021.

Allen, Charlotte. "The Scholars and the Goddess." *The Atlantic.* January 2001.

Encyclopedia.com. "Food in Myth and Legend." Accessed 3/30/2021.

Ferguson, Yuna L., and Kennon M. Sheldon. "Trying to Be Happier Really Can Work: Two Experimental Studies." *The Journal of Positive Psychology* 8, no. 1 (2013): 23–33. doi.org/10.1080/17439760.2012.747000.

Gilbert, Natasha. "The Science of Tea's Mood-Altering Magic." *Nature* 566, S8–S9 (2019): doi:10.1038/d41586-019-00398-1.

Illes, Judika. *Encyclopedia of Spirits: The Ultimate Guide to the Magic of Fairies, Genies, Demons, Ghosts, Gods & Goddesses.* San Francisco: HarperOne, 2009.

Jackson, Jamie. "Corn Mother: The History of Corn." MotherEarthGardener.com. Accessed April 8, 2021.

Keller, Mara Lynn. "Goddess Spirituality" in Leeming, D. A. (ed), *Encyclopedia of Psychology and Religion.* Boston: Springer. doi.org/10.1007/978-1-4614-6086-2_9331.

Legends of American. "Legend of the White Buffalo." Accessed April 6, 2021.

Livius: "Cybele." Livius.org. Accessed December 4, 2020.

Native American Spider Mythology: NativeLanguages.org

Prohom Olson, Danielle. "The Goddess Feasts: The Magic of Gratitude, Pleasure, and Plenty. GatherVictoria.com. Accessed December 1, 2020.

Shaw, Judith. "Rosmerta, the Great Provider—A Celtic Goddess of Abundance." *Feminism and Religion,* 2015.

The Buddhist Centre: TheBuddhistCentre.com

The Sophia Women's Institute, Living Water blog. "Invoking the Goddess: Midsummer Magic and Transformation." TheSophiaWomensInstitute. com. Accessed December 1, 2020.

United Nations of Roma Victrix: UNRV.com

Index

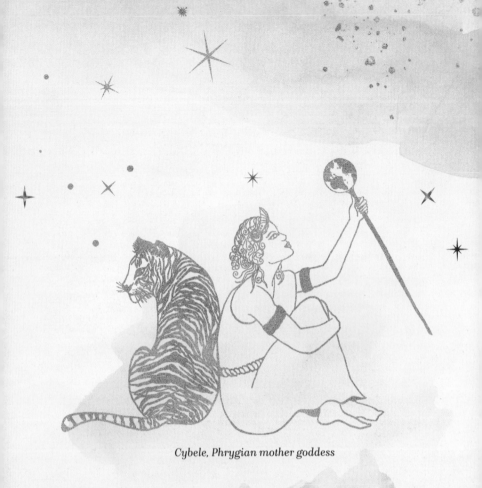

Cybele, Phrygian mother goddess